I0510656

LEGO-BASED THERAPY

LEGO-BASED THERAPY

Current Theory and Practice

DANIEL B. LEGOFF

Universal-Publishers
Irvine • Boca Raton

LEGO-Based Therapy:
Current Theory and Practice

This book and the therapy it describes are not authorized, sponsored,
or endorsed by the LEGO Group.

Copyright © 2023 Daniel B. LeGoff. All rights reserved. No part of this publication
may be reproduced, distributed, or transmitted in any form or by any means, including
photocopying, recording, or other electronic or mechanical methods, without the prior
written permission of the publisher, except in the case of brief quotations embodied in critical
reviews and certain other noncommercial uses permitted by copyright law.

Universal Publishers, Inc.
Irvine & Boca Raton
USA • 2023
www.Universal-Publishers.com

ISBN: 978-1-62734-462-3 (pbk.)
ISBN: 978-1-62734-463-0 (ebk.)
ISBN: 978-1-62734-464-7 (aud.)

For permission to photocopy or use material electronically from this work, please access
www.copyright.com or contact the Copyright Clearance Center, Inc. (CCC) at
978-750-8400. CCC is a not-for-profit organization that provides licenses and registration
for a variety of users. For organizations that have been granted a photocopy license
by the CCC, a separate system of payments has been arranged.

Typeset by Medlar Publishing Solutions Pvt Ltd, India
Cover design by Ivan Popov
Cover illustration by Hannah LeGoff

Library of Congress Cataloging-in-Publication Data

Names: LeGoff, Daniel B., author.
Title: LEGO-based therapy : current theory and practice / Daniel B. LeGoff.
Description: Irvine : Universal-Publishers, [2024] | Includes bibliographical references.
Identifiers: LCCN 2023036772 (print) | LCCN 2023036773 (ebook) |
    ISBN 9781627344623 (pbk.) | ISBN 9781627344630 (ebk.) |
    ISBN 9781627344647 (aud.)
Subjects: LCSH: Play therapy--Methodology. | LEGO toys. |
    Group play therapy--Methodology. | Social skills in children.
Classification: LCC RJ505.P6 L428 2024 (print) | LCC RJ505.P6 (ebook) |
    DDC 618.92/891653--dc23/eng/20230905
LC record available at https://lccn.loc.gov/2023036772
LC ebook record available at https://lccn.loc.gov/2023036773

DEDICATION

To Sir Simon, for his insight and wisdom about the power of empathy, and for being the first to say that letting children design their own therapy using LEGO might, in fact, work.

CONTENTS

INTRODUCTION

As many readers may be familiar, LEGO-based therapy (LBT) started when a few children I was seeing for individual therapy to help with social development showed a common interest in LEGO as a play material. That was over twenty-five years ago and the use of LEGO materials in therapy for children with social development needs has continued to grow and evolve. The fact that the use of LBT has been growing and has adapted to many other settings suggests that it arose from natural, synergistic influences. Initially, it was just two young boys who identified with each other and agreed that it would be fun to play with LEGO together. In doing so, their parents and I realized they were creating an opportunity to improve their own social and communication skills by collaborating on a mutually engaging and fun activity; they were essentially designing their own therapy. Looking back on that experience, it seems to have resulted in a form of interpersonal and cultural synergy, which I recognize now as being at the center of what is missing in the developmental and educational experiences of many children. Engaging in social play is an important activity for all of us, but especially for children since social play is how most children learn about and participate in interpersonal synergy and culture.

In the context of biological and social systems, synergy refers to an organizational dynamic involving communication and collaboration among diverse elements resulting in mutual benefit, growth, and adaptability. The word's etymology is from the Greek, *sun* (together) and *ergon* (work), and later in Latin, *syn* and *ergos* (synergia), meaning, "work together." Latash (2008) has provided a thorough discussion of synergistic dynamics in physiology and movement (kinesiology). The term has also been applied to social collaboration and is now widely used in the social sciences. In addition to its relevance to collaborative human efforts, according to Corning (2022), it is a central characteristic of the evolution and adaptation of all living organisms. All organic systems—from cells to ecosystems—persist because they grow, adapt, and reproduce themselves (von Bertalanffy, 1968a). By contributing diversity and creativity in collaborative ways, individual organisms—including humans—enable species and ecosystems to persist despite harsh and variable environmental conditions. Evolutionary history has shown the importance of synergistic outcomes in the persistence, growth, and adaptability of interpersonal relationships and culture, establishing the basis for larger groups and, eventually, whole civilizations (Corning, 2018; van Schaik & Burkhart, 2011). From the perspective of child development, participating in social and cultural systems is beneficial for both those systems and their participants. The exclusion of individuals from fully participating in each sociocultural system necessarily reduces that system's adaptive fitness and sustainability, while also reducing the benefit for those individuals in terms of their quality of life and opportunities to contribute their unique abilities, skills, experiences, and creativity.

As Meltzoff and his colleagues have shown, the origins of human social relationships are both genetic and learned (Meltzoff, 2007; 2002). As we know from studies of other human traits, such as intelligence, sociality is likely to be distributed normally in human populations, thereby creating a normal bell-shaped distribution, with most people having about average degrees of sociality, with a smaller but still significant number of people being either high or low on sociality. Children with what has been described as the broader autism phenotype (BAP), might also be low on the normally distributed trait of sociality, or innately influenced but developmentally acquired social competence. For many individuals, their early childhood experiences may not support the development of a social self-concept or sense of identity which includes the "like-me," experience of others within their families or close social groups such as peer groups and classrooms. This can create negative cycles of social and cultural isolation leading to unresolved problems of social adjustment that can linger throughout the lifespan, limiting their occupational and sociocultural opportunities and resulting in significant family and individual distress and maladjustment (Posar & Visconti, 2019; Jonsdottir, et al, 2018; Chamak & Bonniau, 2016).

The view that sociality is a trait in humans with a range of levels with both genetic and learned components is supported by extensive research on the concept of the Broader Autism Phenotype (BAP, Kellerman, *et al*, 2019; Ozonoff, *et al*, 2014). According to Tsai, Cebula and Fletcher-Watson's research on siblings of children identified with autistic conditions, the BAP can influence overall adjustment of entire families. The presence of either autistic conditions or the BAP in parents as well as siblings is an important factor influencing the long-term social competence and vocational opportunities in many children who may not have models of interpersonal synergy as an adaptive coping strategy in the home. This is the basis for considerable research and intervention in the general clinical literature on family systems theory (Priest, 2021; Keller & Noone, 2020).

While LBT was not initially identified with a particular model of psychotherapy or child development (LeGoff, 2004), the initial observations and description of this approach were clearly influenced by models of child development which emphasized the importance of social play and peer-mediated learning: social and cultural constructivism (Crawford, 2010; Moll & Tomasello, 2007; Piaget & Inhelder, 1972; Vygotsky, 1967; 1934/1986; 1933/1978); peer-mediated learning and scaffolding (Shvarts & Bakker, 2019; Bruner, 1986; 1973), and integrative developmental neuroscience (Courchesne, 2020; Decety, 2020; Arsalidou & Pascual-Leone, 2016; Decety & Wheatley, 2015; Goncu & Gaskins, 2006; Goncu, 1999). To understand the synergistic outcomes observed in peer-mediated play based on the LBT model (or in any successful play group), it is necessary to recognize the significance of play as a form of learning, creativity, and sociocultural adaptation throughout both recent and remote human history (Grandqvist, 2021; Burghardt, 2015; LaFreniere, 2011; Smith, 2006; Gaskins, Haight & Lancy, 2006). Synergistic dynamics in human genetic and sociocultural evolution have been described as central to the developmental processes underlying both social (Corning, 2018) and language development (DeBoer, 2017, Fitch, Huber & Bugnyar, 2010) as well as in cultural evolution (Grandqvist, 2021; Foley & Lahr, 2011) and creativity (Muthukrishna, *et al*, 2018; Muthukrishna & Heinrich, 2016).

Being willing and able to participate in interpersonal interactions for humans requires a considerable amount of socially mediated learning, which begins in early infancy (Meltzoff, *et al*, 2009; Meltzoff, 2007; 2002; Meltzoff & Moore, 1977), and even before birth (Courchesne, Gazestani, & Lewis, 2020). Children who may have autistic traits such as low sociality or who meet the diagnostic criteria for autistic conditions, do not experience sociocultural synergy—scaffolding and socially-mediated learning of language, culturally-specific forms of play, and socio-emotional norms. For them, their sociocultural context may have more of a negative impact on their development in the form of a simultaneously operating vicious cycle. This inverse of developmental synergy is not a well-established construct, except in the form of vicious circles in mental illness (Reinhard, *et al*, 2020) and chronic pain (Kalso, 2011). Unlike synergistic systems in which the individual elements interact in dynamic, simultaneous ways to maintain the overall viability and robustness of a system, vicious cycles are linear and sequential. Because they are a sequence of effects that maintain a maladaptive pattern, rather than creating an emergent outcome that is distinct from and more than the sum of its parts as in the case of synergy, intervention strategies based on the vicious cycle model tend to emphasize unidimensional interventions which "break the cycle." This approach has rarely been effective, which is why these vicious cycles persist, become chronic, and grow (Sapotka, Houkes & Bosma, 2021; Skuladottir, *et al*, 2020).

Interpersonal synergy refers to ways in which individuals successfully collaborate with each other. Factors which interfere with that process are central to understanding how being autistic can become a limiting or disabling condition. Humans have evolved biologically through genetic and cultural inheritance to have an advanced capacity for collaboration (Corning, 2018; 2011; 2005; 2003). The benefits to society as well as to the life experiences of individuals are clear: modern society relies on cultural collaboration in ever more complex and interdependent ways (Muthukrishna, *et al*, 2018; Muthukrishna & Henrich, 2016). At the same time, synergy is not a universal characteristic of interpersonal interactions, relationships, or sociocultural organizations. While creative, adaptable, and sustainable organizations—like sports teams (Araujo & Davids, 2016; Silva, *et al*, 2013; Stagl, *et al*, 2006), and businesses (Holtzstrom & Anderson, 2021; Someh, Shanks & Davern, 2019; Wartini-Twardowska & Twardowski, 2019; Salmons, Wilson & Strang, 2009)—benefit from synergistic dynamics, maladaptive and destructive sociocultural dynamics also exist. In fact, in Baron Cohen's insightful work on the origins of interpersonal cruelty, or evil in cultural contexts (Baron Cohen, 2011), he emphasized that it results from a breakdown in interpersonal empathy, which can be thought of as a form of emotional synergy.

The emergent or creative element of sharing an emotional experience is empathy, and for a variety of reasons, humans sometimes disconnect from others and then act in ways that undermine the mutual value and benefit of sociocultural collaboration. For that sociocultural context or system, then, interpersonal cruelty or evil is not adaptive, but maladaptive in a persistent and enduring way. Although Baron Cohen used the common term *evil* to describe this phenomenon, I will argue that the work evil or bad, as in being wicked, malicious, or malevolent, focus on the actions of an individual and not on the conditions or system dynamics which can result in persistently maladaptive outcomes for individuals, families, communities, or any other social group. For that reason, I have introduced the word *antergy*, which means literally "working against."

Antergy refers to organizational dynamics in which conflicted values and goals undermine the adaptability of the individual members and the system as a whole. Elements of a system, whether they are individuals, organizations, or subsystems, may work against a common interest or the mutual benefit of other elements of that system resulting in persistent dysfunction, or maladaptive outcomes, such as in a dysfunctional family, a sports team on a losing streak, or a failing business. The underlying problem is often a lack of mutual goals and lack of shared values: parts of a system which do not agree with each other about values or goals will undermine each other as well as the system. At a biological level, invasive species, or invasive cells such as cancers, thrive at the expense rather than for the betterment and adaptive resilience of the host ecosystem or organism. At the societal level, some elements within a civilization or culture may have goals which work against the success of other groups within that civilization, or which attempt to marginalize and undermine diverse individuals. There are so many examples of persistently maladaptive patterns in biological and sociocultural systems, it is somewhat surprising in hindsight that the word antergy does not already exist.

In the case of individuals with low sociality, the BAP, or autistic conditions, antergy involves a combination of factors which simultaneously interfere with adaptive social development, and tend to persist despite focal, break-the-chain types of interventions. Some educators and therapists do not seem to be aware of the benefit of interpersonal synergy—which relies on diversity and inclusion for the adaptive success of sociocultural systems—but work against the interests of diverse individuals by identifying their struggles as forms of pathology, rather than viewing them as potentially adaptive and beneficial contributors to their sociocultural systems. Unlike parents who intuitively and naturally value and support their children's unique, creative contributions, some communities, schools, and even forms of therapy, advocate for elimination of diversity and implementation of uniformity by imposing arbitrary standards of conduct, appearance, interests, and modes of self-expression. Rather than being flexibly adaptive to support synergistic growth, these approaches tend to reduce degrees of freedom and result in persisting forms of antergy: maladaptive outcomes that supported by those elements within a sociocultural system which do not share the same values as the children and families they purport to be helping.

Antergy, in that sense, can also be defined and observed as operations which reduce rather than increase the degrees of freedom within a system. From the point of view of development and learning, any organism gains internal degrees of freedom when its internal system—biological and/or cognitive—can choose or determine the values of relevant variables in the system in which that organism participates. While synergistic operations and experiences increase the degrees of freedom in which an organism can adaptively participate, antergistic operations reduce those degrees of freedom and the mutual benefit of organisms and their ecosystems. A common and familiar example would be a persisting drought in an ecosystem which reduces the degrees of freedom in terms of adaptive actions of the organisms in that ecosystem by limiting their access to water, causing a maladaptive shrinking and rapid decline of the ecosystem, faster than predicted by the decrease in water alone. Another example is overly rigid and conservative cultures in which religious beliefs, self-expression and individual identity are restricted. These systems inevitably remain dysfunctional and isolated rather than integrated with other sociocultural systems and supporting new, creative systems. Political regimes which suppress individuality and self-expression, and which enforce conformity and reduce individual freedoms are another example.

In social constructivism, individual children learn and adapting within a sociocultural and historical context. As is evident in various forms of developmental psychopathology, the results can be either synergistic and adaptive, or antergistic and maladaptive, for both the individuals and their sociocultural systems. While synergy is a dynamic that reflects mutual benefit, antergy reflects mutual harm. Rather than thinking of child development as a linear sequence of events, the constructivist model views children as active and creative participants in complex historical, interpersonal, and cultural systems. Understanding children, then, requires us to consider the dynamic systems that are part of them—bodies and brains, cognition, emotions, values—and around them—sociocultural environment—which work together. Children do not just learn from the world around them; they creatively contribute to it. That is how sociocultural systems themselves can adapt and persist across generations: they are synergistic. When a child is kept from participating in sociocultural systems for some reason, their development will be negatively affected, as will the systems in which they might participate. In the case of antergy, however, there are maladaptive factors which sustain and amplify that negative impact on both the child and their sociocultural systems.

To understand how antergistic dynamics operate for autistic individuals in society, it is important to understand constructivism and the reciprocal nature of child development and sociocultural systems. The "like me" dynamic described by Meltzoff and his colleagues (Meltzoff, *et al*, 2009, Meltzoff, 2007) appears to be the developmental origin of intuitive social cognition and theory of mind (Brooks & Meltzoff, 2015; Haxby, Hoffman & Gobbini, 2002) for most children. This phenomenon is present in early infancy, and results in interpersonal attachment and social identity formation. These in turn are prerequisites for increasing a child's attending to and learning from their social environment, relative to their physical environment (Guo, *et al*, 2017). The first phase of attachment and identification has a long-lasting impact on the child's self-concept which we might call *anthropocentrism*, which is a characteristic of the human species which is observable throughout history and in every culture. This is a tendency to value and promote our own species and our sociocultural systems at the expense of other species and other systems, such as ecosystems or even the entire planet.

Anthropocentrism is evident in early infancy in the tendency to focus on and sustain attention to human-like features and culturally relevant events, which is a type of anthropocentric tropism (anthropotropism). A tropism is an innate or instinctive tendency to maintain contact with a range of events identified with an external source, such as the way plants move to expose their photosynthetic cells towards the sun (phototropism). Plants also grow in ways influenced by the available sunlight in their immediate surroundings, a biological phenomenon known as photomorphogenesis. In that sense, typical human infants are born with an innate tendency to both orient towards their social environment (anthropotropism) and to develop in ways which allow them to maintain contact with other people and participate in human systems (anthropomorphogenesis). For children diagnosed with autistic conditions, or those with the BAP, however, there are gene-environment dynamics which show less evidence of these instinctive dynamics, and in the long-run result in less evidence of anthropocentrism, or sociality.

This may seem to be offering a biological theory for something that is obvious and common sense, but in fact, our understanding of the dynamic operations of biological systems within humans as organisms and in their interactions with their ecosystems is a relatively new field within science. Although von Bertalanffy described general systems theory as a model for understanding organisms and their niches, replacing the standard linear cause-effect models, in the middle of the last century (von Bertalanffy, 1950, 1934), it was not until much later that theorists began to understand and explore the implications of systems theory for human systems (Elwell, 2013; Brody, 1973; Laszlo, 1972a; 1972b; 1969). It has only been very recently that we have begun to examine the important variables influencing the dynamic interactions of organic and sociocultural systems in child development (Guralnick, 2019; Perone & Simmering, 2017; Spencer, Perone & Buss, 2011).

In short, if we think about children as dynamic organic systems who are active and creative participants in the physical and sociocultural systems around them, we are less likely to mistakenly assume that simplistic, top-down interventions such as are offered by operant conditioning theory (aka, applied behavior analysis), will be of benefit rather than harm. One of the important insights about children who have lower innate sociality levels is that this is not by itself a problem for that child, their family, or their larger sociocultural systems. That is the point of view promoted by the neurodiversity movement (Chapman, 2021; Leadbitter, *et al*, 2021; den Houting, 2019). This issue has been discussed elsewhere (LeGoff, 2023). Historically, individuals with diverse and unique developmental pathways and life experiences have always been important to the adaptability and richness of sociocultural systems. In recent times, however, there has been an increased emphasis on professional scrutiny of children due to a combination of factors such as laws ensuring equal access to and benefit from public services including education—such the Americans with Disabilities Act (ADA), and the Individuals with Disabilities Education Act (IDEA)—and the promotion of autism as a diagnosis and advocacy for early childhood developmental and educational services. This increased focus on atypicality and/or low sociality as signs of developmental pathology may be responsible for many of the problems faced by autistic individuals, rather than the other way around.

In this context, one of the biggest problems with increased professional scrutiny of infants and children—especially by those with specialized training who may themselves have professional and economic motivations for identifying children and families who are candidates for receiving their services—is the lack of understanding of the long-term outcomes of developmental and educational interventions. Rather than allowing existing sociocultural systems, such as classrooms and communities, to organically adapt to a child's unique needs, the emphasis on top-down behavioral and psychopharmacological interventions results in identifying the problem as the child needing to be fixed. This emphasis alone can initiate complex sociocultural dynamics at many levels which can sustain and magnify maladaptive outcomes. Societies with advanced child health, family support, and special education also have widely accessible media and information systems. Misinformation and distorted beliefs can undermine large scale adaptive responses to developmental differences and even initiate maladaptive ones. These maladaptive processes for the individual and their sociocultural systems are *antergistic*; they are not simply due to the absence of social synergy or stalling of adaptive developmental processes but are maladaptive and harmful processes.

Many of the negative life experiences of autistic individuals attest to the potential for poor outcomes and even harmful, antergistic ones. A number of long-term outcome studies have shown that having autistic traits can lead to significant problems in adulthood with social isolation (Davis & Crompton, 2021; Maitland, *et al*, 2021; Cage, Monaco & Newell, 2018; Farley, *et al*, 2018, Heninger & Taylor, 2013; Howlin & Moss, 2012; Farley *et al*, 2009), anxiety (Andrews, *et al*, 2022), and depressed mood (Maitland, *et al*, 2021). These are not characteristics of being autistic or having a developmental disability, *per se*, but may be the results of psychosocial stressors and withdrawal from negative social influences (Maitland, *et al*, 2021; Lawson, Mathys & Rees, 2017; Esbenson, *et al*, 2010) and unemployment or under-employment (Solomon, 2020; Frank, *et al*, 2018; Ohl, *et al*, 2017). There appears to be evidence of reiterative feedback loops ("vicious cycles,") involving both autistic children and their parents and other family members (Sosnowy, Silverman & Shattuck, 2017; Chamak & Bonniau, 2016; Keenan, *et al*, 2016). In this regard, there is an emerging literature on individuals who have attempted to "camouflage" their autism by behaving consistently with social expectations and norms, but for whom social activities and fitting into typical sociocultural environments is experienced as stressful, anxiety-provoking, and depressing

(Hull, *et al*, 2021; Cage & Troxell-Whitman, 2019). For most autistic adults, persisting difficulties with social adjustment, employment, and physical health are neither considered nor addressed by current childhood education or clinical interventions (Weir, *et al*, 2021a & 2021b).

Unfortunately, due to the over-emphasis on behavioral treatments and behavioral outcomes in autism services, addressing anxiety and depression as emerging issues in autistic individuals has received little attention in the clinical literature (Wood, *et al*, 2009, Mesibov, 1992). There is also emerging evidence that intensive ABA-based interventions may have their own negative social, emotional, educational, and vocational impact on autistic individuals (Sandoval-Norton, Shkedy & Shkedy, 2021; Sandoval-Norton & Shkedy, 2019). The experience of many individuals and their family members who have undergone ABA-based autism interventions is that these prolonged and invasive procedures did not yield benefits which justified the personal and financial costs (Jonsdottir, *et al*, 2018; Chamak & Bonniau, 2016). Despite years of prolonged and daily behavioral intervention, many autistic individuals do not achieve common adaptive milestones like completing post-secondary education (Frank, *et al*, 2018), getting a job (Solomon, 2020; Ohl, *et al*, 2017; Baldwin, Costley & Warren, 2014), living independently (Anderson, *et al*, 2014), and learning to drive (Myers, *et al*, 2019; Wilson, *et al*, 2018; Lindsay, 2017). Due to the exclusive focus on short-term, observable outcomes in behavioral programs, long-term adaptive outcomes are either ignored or assumed to be the responsibility of the children and their families. The unproved, and demonstrably mistaken assumption made by behavior analysts—and other educators and therapists influenced by their methods—is that changing a child's behavior using operant conditioning techniques in any given setting will carry-over, or have generalized effects, in terms of adaptive functioning in other settings later.

This mistaken view is derived from the use of operant conditioning techniques developed in animal laboratories and then applied to individuals diagnosed with autism and other developmental disabilities in highly controlled institutional environments (Ferster, 1961; Ferster & DeMyer, 1961). After demonstrating some degree of behavior change using operant conditioning with human subjects, advocates of using Skinnerian operant conditioning methods with human children such as Ivar Lovaas (Lovaas, 1981; Lovaas, *et al*, 1974; Lovaas, *et al*, 1973), achieved widespread popularity. These studies on early intensive behavioral interventions (EIBI), which proposed using highly controlled, adult-directed learning trials with preschoolers for forty hours per week or more, demonstrated increased rates of compliance with tasks intended to demonstrate classroom readiness skills (sitting still, attending to verbal commands, object-action imitation, verbal imitation, object, and picture matching, pointing to indicate verbal comprehension, etc.).

Although Lovaas and his colleagues reported unprecedented levels of improvement in classroom readiness in preschoolers, and even showed improvements in IQ scores (Lovaas, 1993; McEachin, Smith & Lovaas, 1993; Lovaas, 1987), the procedures used were viewed as bordering on inhumane, and these outcomes were not able to be replicated. Just as importantly, though, there was no evidence that the children who participated in these studies had similar characteristics, or long-term meaningful benefits. Just as Skinner had not demonstrated any meaningful benefit of his operant conditioning experiments for the rats and pigeons who participated, Lovaas and his colleagues seemed to have no interest in the life outcomes for the participants in their EIBI studies. Despite the obvious flaws of this approach, there has been an accelerating rate of growth in ABA-based clinical and educational services including a rapid expansion of the number of graduates from behavior analysis programs. These programs have eclipsed and even replaced the roles of child psychologists and special education teachers, despite the board-certification programs in behavior analysis offering no training in either child psychology or special education.

The main flaw with ABA as a model for understanding and supporting development and education for autistic children is that its theory and methods necessarily reduce identity, culture, play, and sociocultural systems to behavior and operant conditioning. Human evolutionary sociocultural history is not reducible to the influences of positive reinforcement. Behavior analytic models do not consider many other factors which are integral components of both child development and human history, such as human brain development, family dynamics, interpersonal relationships, creativity, cognitive development, and symbolic communication. It is these complex areas of sociocultural evolution and development which are the primary hurdles for autistic individuals. The experience of life as an autistic individual is the perspective that should be the primary focus in strategies used to help autistic individuals lead more fulfilling lives. Ironically, behavior analysts intentionally ignore the subjective experiences of individuals which they understand as being irrelevant to their behavior. Due to the biases of radical behaviorism, ABA-based services are not only ineffective as interventions but inherently dehumanizing (LeGoff, 2023).

LEGO-based therapy developed in a synergistic and adaptive way from the participation of its individual members, reflecting both individual and shared values and goals. The initial outcome studies (LeGoff & Sherman, 2006; LeGoff, 2004) did not focus on immediate, observable changes in behavior, but on the participants' social motivation and social competence with peers in natural settings. This emphasis on improvement in social and communication domains of adaptive functioning was what made LBT quickly popular among the children and parents, and subsequently to gain favor among an international group of educators and therapists. Parents and educators are intuitively aware that the greatest hurdles for autistic individuals involve social adjustment and the capacity to participate in sociocultural systems. It is these systems which have historically supported human civilization, including individuals' benefiting from and contributing to their families, workplaces, communities, and societies. While operant conditioning and behavioral compliance may be helpful to teachers in teaching standardized curricula in structured classrooms, daily life for most adults involves self-initiated participation in sociocultural systems; and that is not the result of positive reinforcement, but of social motivation, affiliation, identification, and shared accomplishment.

In addition to being an outdated reductionistic and deterministic theory, radical behaviorism is inconsistent with central human values which are also essential to all living organisms: diversity, inclusion, self-determination, creativity, and synergy. Typically developing children follow a path towards active and creative participation in the shared accomplishment and mutually beneficial synergy of sociocultural systems. The offspring of many species, including humans, exhibit typical play as a way of learning about and creatively contributing to the diversity and adaptability of their culturally specific social norms, methods of communication, and technologies (Goncu & Gaskins, 2006). Autistic children, or those with the BAP, show diminished social attachment and identification in early infancy (Ashmawi & Hammoda, 2022; Zwaigenbaum, *et al*, 2015; Turati, *et al*, 2013; Ozonoff, *et al*, 2010; Webb & Jones, 2009; van Ijzendoorn, *et al*, 2007; Toth, *et al*, 2006; Dawson, *et al*, 2004). While these prenatal or early infant differences in sociality may initially be neurobiological and possibly genetic, their consequences can have a rapidly escalating cascade effect on sociocultural learning, family functioning, and adaptability (Martin, *et al*, 2020; Keller, 2018; Groh, *et al*, 2017; Winston & Chicot, 2016; Grzadinski, *et al*, 2014; Rutgers, *et al*, 2004).

The literature on early identification and intervention for autistic children and their families has shifted in recent years from an emphasis on early diagnosis and behavioral intervention, to early identification of at-risk infants and preventative or preemptive strategies (Whitehouse, 2017). This approach emphasizes the use of parent-mediated play-based strategies to improve social attachment, social communication, and social identity formation in infants at risk for autistic features or the BAP (Green, *et al*, 2022; Whitehouse, *et al*, 2021; Green, 2020; Whitehouse, *et al*, 2019; Green, *et al*, 2018; Green, *et al*, 2017; Green, *et al*, 2013). The outcome literature on parent-mediated social communication interventions in early infancy has included both standardized intervention models (Green, *et al*, 2022) as well as randomized control-group studies (Green, *et al*, 2017), which are models of outcome research not used by ABA researchers. While these researchers are showing some important findings in humane, non-invasive, and cost-effective interventions, these strategies are not in widespread use, and many infants at risk will not have access to advanced early detection methods.

In addition to some limitations with accessibility, the preventative or preemptive models described above focus primarily on attachment, play, and social communication which can have long-term effects on social development, but there are also likely to be sociocultural development and learning challenges later in childhood and adolescence which ABA does not address. In other words, although this model offers considerable promise for improving early social identification and attachment in infants at risk for autistic social adjustment difficulties, older children and adolescents with autistic features may still need additional support and learning opportunities to achieve social competence. Many children with autistic features are better adjusted at home, and in other settings such as the classroom, where the social environment is less challenging, more accepting, and where they have access to adult support.

The LBT model introduces children at gradual, self-regulated levels to social and communication challenges like those they encounter in educational, vocational, and community environments. The goals for children in LBT involve creative participation in a sociocultural system. It is presented as a fun and self-affirming opportunity—which is the way most children experience sociocultural environments—not as a challenge or as an adult-directed intervention. The main activity of the group involves different forms of LEGO play—from pre-building activities to advanced, creative use of LEGO sets in animated film production—which the children themselves identify as an activity in which they accel. For many children who do not have much experience with or even interest in LEGO, the group activities allow them to create opportunities to share their idiosyncratic interests, which are often compatible with LEGO-based creative activities. The important developmental gains supported by LBT include:

- social identification with peers and increased motivation to participate in peer-based activities.
- positive, self-affirming experiences of joint accomplishment, shared creativity, and synergistic outcomes.
- self-initiated participation in gradually increasing levels of social collaboration, communication, and leadership.
- insight and internalization of the interpersonal and communication dynamics of sociocultural environments which are immediately relevant and useful in other sociocultural settings.
- peer-mediated acceptance, support, and encouragement of self-expression and creativity in joint accomplishment and culturally relevant activities.

The values which underly the theory and methods of LBT derive from an understanding of the core principles of organic systems and the central importance of life experience. These include:

- Diversity and inclusion, as opposed to compliance and conformity.
- Self-determination versus learned helplessness.
- Synergistic creativity through participation in sociocultural systems, rather than simply fitting in, sharing, or taking turns.
- Improving social and communication self-efficacy and interpersonal competence, as opposed to task accomplishment and reactance against adult-led activities.
- Personally meaningful experiences and social connections with peers, instead of *naturalistic* and adult-directed experiences.

The next two chapters were published in LeGoff (2023) and are replicated here so that the reader has access to these summaries of the development of

LBT and its popularization. This topic has also been previously reviewed and discussed in detail in a previous book, LeGoff (2017). This book is intended as a more in-depth and updated version of LeGoff, *et al* (2014). As noted above, that manual was written long before it was published, and there has been considerable growth in the LBT methodology and culture since then. The most important differences between the current overview of LBT and that of LeGoff, *et al* (2014), are the following:

- The theoretical rationale involving the importance of childhood experiences of interpersonal and sociocultural synergy for the development of social competence, creativity, and participation in sociocultural systems has been developed, scrutinized, and presented in various publications and workshops.
- The influence of ABA-based strategies has been removed, consistent with the view that ABA is derived from the radical behaviorist methods of instrumental or operant conditioning which is incompatible with synergistic systems models of child development both theoretically and pragmatically.
- The structure and activities of the groups themselves have grown and evolved to include much more diversity of roles, an increased emphasis on social communication rather than LEGO activities themselves, and an increased emphasis on play and creativity rather than adult-directed activities.
- There has been a broad range of studies on LBT from culturally and professionally diverse research perspectives.
- The LBT methodology has been utilized with populations other than autistic children and adolescents to include a broader range of social and communication goals and needs.
- LEGO itself—the corporation and its products—have changed and grown considerably over the years. Notably, the LEGO Corporation has facilitated the expansion of the non-profit LEGO Foundation, which not only supports research and training on child development and play (Liu, *et al*, 2017), they have supported research on implementation of LBT (Wright, *et al*, 2017).
- Finally, there has been an opportunity for me and other providers to get feedback about the LBT experience from those who participated in the therapy over the years, and who are now young adults who are able to reflect on their experiences and how LBT has influenced their lives.

CHAPTER 1

THE DEVELOPMENT OF LEGO-BASED THERAPY

It was just about thirty years ago that I thought about starting a LEGO group for autistic children. I have written about the details of that experience elsewhere (LeGoff, 2017; LeGoff, *et al*, 2014; 2011; 2010; LeGoff & Sherman, 2006; LeGoff, 2004), but some of the details about it are worth reviewing in this context since they shed light on what seems to have been a successful form of interpersonal synergy. The most important aspect of it from my point of view was that both the idea and then the process of setting up and running the LEGO-based therapy groups was accomplished entirely by the participants themselves. As I have said and written elsewhere, I just paid for the LEGO and the kids did the rest. What I mean by "the rest," is basically everything it took for them to convince me to make the groups happen so that they could participate, collaborate, and create together. Although the LEGO groups have since become a more formal evidence-based therapy model, what guided its development was playful collaboration, and the results were naturally synergistic.

There has been considerable research on play-based intervention for autistic children, including numerous reviews which offer guidelines for effective and ethical implementation of these strategies (Gibson, Pritchard & de Lemos, 2021; Moody & Laugeson, 2020; Gallo-Lopez & Rubin, 2011; Hull, 2011; Reichow & Volkmar, 2010). In their extensive review and synthesis of the research literature on play-based social and communication development strategies, Gibson, *et al* (2021) conclude:

Overall, the data highlights the importance of multi-disciplinary approaches in this field. Congruent with a multi-disciplinary approach, we also found that play-based interventions frequently target multiple outcomes—an approach that makes sense given the pervasive nature of social communication difficulties in autism. Social play skills were the largest single type of outcome target, measured in 16.5% of studies. This ties in with the increasing recognition that play is a crucial tool for supporting learning and development, particularly in social domains (p. 20).

This meta-analytic study revealed many weaknesses or gaps in the research literature on social and communication interventions for autistic children, with the bulk of evidence-based research being done within the adult-directed or behaviorist framework. They point out that while it is widely accepted that typical children develop social and communication skills through self-directed and peer-mediated playful interactions, creating conditions in which these features are replicated and are monitored and measured in terms of their impact, is more complicated than it might seem. In other words, getting typical children together to work on social and communication skills involves minimal effort; we adults just need to give them a safe place, some play materials, and then stay out of their way. Trying to design something similar for autistic children who do not normally initiate playful interaction and communication with peers, and who may not share common interests or preferred play activities with other children, is much more difficult. The complications also include finding some way to objectively assess progress in relevant domains which can justify the method, while also not interfering with the process (i.e., staying out of their way).

The LEGO Club, Then and Now. The origins of LEGO-based therapy (LBT) were synergistic in the sense that there were diverse contributors who both benefited from and contributed to the process, a hierarchy of decision-making, and an outcome that was both not predicted by and greater than its components. The initial impetus in starting to use LEGO in therapy at all came from the inadvertent observation that several the children I was seeing in my outpatient practice showed a greater interest in building with the LEGO materials in my playroom during therapy sessions than other play or expressive materials. They also seemed more willing to engage with me interactively and through both verbal and nonverbal communication when the therapeutic focus included LEGO. In addition to this preference for LEGO as a playful, expressive, and creative material, the children with autistic conditions also often noticed and commented on the LEGO creations that were on display nearby on the bookshelves or table surfaces.

This was an important observation for me since I had noticed that autistic children rarely noticed evidence of other children's activities in the room, such as drawings, clay sculptures, or sand tray activity. They would not point to a child's drawing or a plasticene sculpture and ask who had done it, or even notice and ask about the photos of my own children in the room. They did, however, notice and become curious about the LEGO creations, both sets and freestyle, and they would ask about the children who had made them. They asked what their names were, and how old they were, and how often they came to see me. They asked me why I thought the other child had chosen that design, and even what that child's interests were, and if they were going to do more LEGO creating. They also asked if the other children had seen or commented on their LEGO creations. This social interest, perspective-taking, and evidence of theory of mind about other children who were not even in the room was a marked change in social reasoning and sociality for autistic children. It led me to think that they might be identifying with those other children based on this common interest and affinity for LEGO which led to a "like me," experience, as Meltzoff (2007; 2002; Meltzoff, *et al*, 2009) has described it. In other words, they seemed to be expressing a sense of identification and affiliation with others because of this shared area of interest and value. It was as if they sensed that these other children must be like them because they shared this value for an external system, the system of LEGO.

As I have documented elsewhere, the idea of working with two children together using LEGO came from a single event in which two boys met in the waiting room of my practice while their parents were at the reception desk. They had both brought LEGO creations with them. They did not introduce themselves to each other, but they showed a mutual initiating of joint attention, and sharing of verbal communication about their interest in LEGO. They also talked about some other interests, including anime and space exploration, which inspired one of the boys to say to me later, "You know, Dr. Dan, that kid is from my planet." That confirmed for me that there had been a spark of recognition, identification, and a sense of affiliation between the two, which was atypical for both. I had immediately envisioned trying to capitalize on that shared interest to create an opportunity for them to participate in joint therapy focused on improving their social reciprocity, communication, and problem-solving, but I also knew both boys well enough to predict that they would probably be content to engage in LEGO-based parallel play, with minimal direct social interaction or communication.

I recall thinking about how I could get the two boys to collaborate on a project and be motivated to get over whatever differences or difficulties they might have by directly sharing a favorite activity which they both enjoyed doing on their own. I had some experience already using LEGO materials in a collaborative way in individual therapy sessions in which I would intrude into the process by asking questions or giving suggestions when a child needed help with something they were working on, but that was somewhat annoying to them rather than helpful and fun. I had noticed, though, that they often seemed to appreciate it when I would find a certain piece for them, whether it was a piece in a LEGO set, or just a piece that they wanted to help complete a freestyle creation they were putting together. It was also a good opportunity to help them work on functional communication by getting them to describe the pieces they wanted, including the shape, size, color, and function of the pieces, and what they needed them for. We could go back and forth for quite a long time just talking about LEGO pieces, what might work or not, and what we were able to find in my small collection of spare parts.

One of the more obviously exciting experiences for my LEGO fan clients was getting a new set to build. We would look at LEGO magazines and catalogues—this was before internet shopping—and talk about that they might want to have me get as an addition to the LEGO materials in the playroom. The type of communication and the choices of LEGO set were different for each child, but the process was equally thrilling for them, and there was a sense of collaboration in the planning for a new set. I would sometimes call an order with the child, and they would help me get a representative on the phone, give them the set code, and my credit card information. The entire process was something that might be considered tedious—ordering parts on the phone from a catalogue—but it was LEGO, which made it exciting. Then we would wait for the set to show up, and quite often there would be more than one child waiting for the same set that I had promised to order. Then when it finally showed up, the group had a whole session or two to assemble it.

During those sessions, we shared the tasks as much as possible, and made sure that we would not lose any pieces, or the instructions, and that we completed the set methodically and accurately. We carefully opened the box and emptied the parts into plastic lunch trays (which I had purchased at a dollar store for that purpose), looked at the usual advertising that came with it, and then got out the directions. Before we got to the directions and the building, we would sort through the pieces and organize them a bit, admiring any novel or unfamiliar bricks or special pieces like cloth, or human accessories (weapons, tools, headgear, capes), unusually large pieces, transparent plastic, stickers, magnets, and certainly anything battery-operated. At that time, the instruction pages did not include the pieces that were being added on each page, so we had to scan the pages together to see what new and which piece was still needed to be found on the trays. The larger sets with over a hundred pieces took a lot of tray space to organize and lay out the pieces so that we could find them efficiently.

The child was usually allowed to start assembling the pieces—often it was the mini-figs that were sorted out and assembled first—but we would look at the directions together, and I would offer them the correct pieces only when they identified them accurately, either by pointing to them in the directions or by labeling them verbally. Depending on how that was going, I would often emphasize the need for them to communicate by giving them the wrong piece so they would have to correct me and be more specific—"No, Dr. Dan! It has an angle this way, and there are four bumps,"—or I would purposely lose my focus and they would have to direct me back to the task—"Dr. Dan, you're not paying attention. You must help me find the pieces." At some point, I would ask them to let me take over doing the assembling and they would take charge of sorting and finding the right pieces. Again, I would often make newcomer mistakes and put the pieces in the wrong place or not know how to do the next step at all, so the child would have to help me with verbal directions, gestures, and pointing at the directions. When collaborating on building LEGO sets, we found there were many things to communicate about, and many ways to communicate about them.

When I first asked the two boys to come to a session together, I made sure I had a new set that they both were anticipating building, and I planned to have the three of us build it together. Luckily, there was a natural division of labor that resulted from the LEGO set building process itself: reading the directions, finding the pieces, and assembling them. Luckily, those tasks were all interdependent and could be done simultaneously and with a considerable amount of shared attention and shared accomplishment. It was also fortuitous that the process involved many repetitive but varied tasks, so there was stability and variability or flexibility: building LEGO sets has a certain format and stable process, but it is also different for each new set. Each set contains many familiar and new pieces which follow certain dynamics and principles of form and function, and each step in building a set or a freestyle creates an opportunity for collaboration, communication, joint attention, and joint accomplishment. I did not impose my sense of division of labor with the boys, but we agreed that if there was only one set to build it made sense to divide the tasks horizontally and each participate throughout, rather than just taking turns at working on it or each doing about a third of the project in turns. We also agreed that we could switch roles, from doing the building to looking at the directions, or from looking at the directions, to finding the pieces.

Collaboratively building LEGO sets together was the beginning of what became a long tradition of shared enjoyment and communication, and it was clear right from the first set that we were also building a sense of identity together. At the second collaborative session, we decided together to refer to the separate roles in set-building as being an engineer (following the set directions), a parts-supplier (sorting and finding the pieces), and a builder (assembling the pieces). What we also spontaneously noticed was that when we shared the task this way, building a set took much less time and effort. It is much harder and more time consuming to try to read directions and find the added pieces, then look for them on the tray, and then go back to the partly assembled set and add the piece in the right spot and in the correct orientation. When each of us could focus on a simpler task, we were also able to overlap our actions a bit to help make the other's tasks easier and more efficient. The engineer could show the directions to the part supplier who could line up or even do pre-assembly on some parts (e.g., putting plastic windows into frames, or putting tires on wheel rims), and then hand them to builder just when they needed them, while the engineer showed them where the pieces went in the image and on the set itself.

LEGO bricks have a natural hierarchy as objects, parts of larger objects, functional elements, and as symbols. LEGO sets and freestyle creations have a structure like a language, but they are also tangible, physical objects in themselves. In this way they have both practical, physical properties, and they are representational and can be used to subjectively express something (Nathan Sawaye, the LEGO artist, often discusses this aspect of his work). In the room, working on building LEGO together, these distinct elements of the system blurred together. For instance, after set building, the boys often wanted to either modify a set they had built, or they wanted to do some freestyle building. I was happy to facilitate either activity, but I maintained that we should continue to work together, and not just drifting apart and doing our own thing. The boys did not disagree with me, and they seemed to intuitively understand that there was something valuable about us building together which was more than building on our own, that it was somehow a special experience.

It did not take long for other children, especially those who had an interest in LEGO, to notice the results of what the three of us, Aaron, Sam, and I, (the fictitious names I gave them in my previous book which described their involvement in the development of LBT) were up to. In the book (LeGoff, 2017), the next boys to join us were Evan, Jonathan, and Keith. They had been excited to see the new LEGO sets and the clever freestyle creations emerging on the bookshelves and tabletops in the LEGO corner of my playroom. Many children would come into that room and occupy themselves with dress-up materials, or the sand tray, or jumping around on the little trampoline onto foam blocks, but the growing number of elementary school aged kids who were both identified as autistic and who were fascinated by LEGO continued to grow. At first, there were just a couple of other kids who saw that there were new sets and freestyle creations appearing in the playroom, and they were curious about those LEGO and the kids who were building them. They identified with them, and wanted to meet them, but what was just as important to me was that they also wanted to be met. The children I was working with who were fascinated by LEGO felt that this was a valuable fascination, which included them.

When autistic children who played with LEGO at home saw that other children who came to my office also played with LEGO, at home and in my playroom, they understood that those children valued LEGO building as a creative skill. There was a reciprocal appreciation for that skillset and knowledge base, which is a precursor for culture. Being good at LEGO not only meant that these other children had a common interest and shared a value for that activity, but they were also likely to value them. Many of these children had never identified with and shared enough interests with other children to experience being valued or admired by them. The promise of being valued by someone for some aspect of yourself that is just part of who you are, not an achievement or a struggle, but simply knowing that someone else values you for who you are, was a powerful experience for them. Not only were these kids cool because they played with LEGO, but that might also be a reciprocal feeling.

Those children also sensed that there was something special happening in the playroom, which was more than just events happening in the playroom when they were not there. They wanted to be a part of the action. I had seen this kind of attraction in my own children and in many other children with whom I worked who were not autistic: the attraction of group play. Not being part of LEGO Club was like not getting invited to the birthday party, or not being on the team, for children who had previously never liked birthday parties and could not have cared less about being on teams. When autistic children understand how the LEGO system works, they understand that they can represent an infinite number of objects and events with it, and they are not required to follow sociocultural conventions or interpersonal norms to do it; it is something they sense they are going to be good at. The LEGO system comes with its own rules, and they are communicated visually, and they have a synergistic quality: how you build LEGO is why you build LEGO, just like playing a sport, or doing anything else you enjoy for its own sake. A hobby can be a calling to some people, as it is to many adult fans of LEGO (AFOLs). In the LEGO Club, though, there was an unspoken yet clear understanding that this was a LEGO Club, a place where like-minded children could meet and do what they love to do together.

CHAPTER 2

THE BROADER IMPACT OF LEGO-BASED THERAPY

The first encouraging news I got about the idea of using LEGO as the basis for group therapy came from the kids themselves. They showed up for every session early and were usually excited to be at my office and eager to start. They never seemed to wonder why there was a LEGO Club at my office, they just knew that it was fun, the LEGO was cool, and so were the other kids. The next good news I got was from their parents, teachers, and other school staff who had noticed an immediate qualitative change in most of the participants. They seemed more willing to communicate about their experiences in general but were eager to tell their teachers and friends about LEGO Club, and about their projects. They were also reported to be showing improvements in fine motor skills, and were less irritable, rigid, and self-absorbed. The final good news I got was when I started hearing from other professionals that they wanted to find out more about LEGO Club and why it seemed to be so popular with the kids and their families.

It was not until I had collaborated with several public and private schools and had a long waiting list of children waiting for openings in one of the seven or eight groups that I was running each week by then. Eventually, other psychologists, speech pathologists, OTs, and even psychiatrists came to visit the LEGO Club, and would sit in on groups. The group members were always happy to tell visitors about LEGO Club and show them their projects and the projects of the other groups. Most of them and their parents who visited the room at times to get an idea of what it might be about, rarely needed much more than a few quick explanations. They were told the children were chosen to have similar developmental and age levels and were working on similar social development issues. Each group was held once per week for about an hour and a half, and the groups were open-ended and relatively unstructured. There was a level system, and the group members themselves decided on each other's level. The group members were not allowed to do individual projects—they could do those at home and bring in pictures—the club was for group projects.

My therapy assistants and I were there to help the group members communicate and interact effectively, and to help solve administrative problems, or irresolvable conflicts. Otherwise, the LEGO Club was pretty much up to them, including the choice of rules, and the enforcement of them. They also were responsible for reminding each other about the "rules of cool," which were ways that they could be helpful and supportive to each other. From their perspective, LEGO Club was fun because they got to participate in building and creating projects that were bigger and more interesting than they could build by themselves—the group had an interpersonal synergistic dynamic, which was a new experience to most of them—and they got to have friends. Most of the group members' parents shared names and numbers or email addresses with each other, and some even started LEGO Club websites or social media sites and they uploaded digital photos of the projects and the LEGO Club birthday parties and graduation ceremonies. The group members supported each other through stressful times, and they typically shared spontaneously about their difficulties at school or at home, including personal losses and life changes.

The first generation of LEGO Club group took place at a few locations in Honolulu, in the mid to late 1990's, and it was in the early 2000's that my family and I moved from Hawaii to New Jersey. During that transition, I was able to publish the first LEGO-based therapy outcome study which was based on the data I had collected in Hawaii. That was the first step in a series of steps that led to a growing awareness of the LEGO Club model. I was soon hearing from other therapists from all over the world who had read my article published in 2004 and were able to pick up enough from just that article to start their own clubs. The model was both user friendly and obvious in some ways—autistic children building LEGO collaboratively just made sense, and most people just got it and went with it—but it also had a lot of nuances, and little decisions about which I was getting a lot of questions. Choosing the materials, the lay out of the room, the storage bins, the age of the children, the number of children, and the mix of children; the business aspects of it, like how much to charge, and whether to use insurance or private pay (health insurance does cover it, as a form of group therapy), and whether the groups could be run in school settings or just clinics.

The first time I met Simon Baron Cohen (now Sir Simon) was when he was invited as the keynote speaker at a conference in Philadelphia. He was there to talk about his new book, *The Essential Difference*, and I gave one of my first public talks about LEGO therapy. I asked audience members volunteer to come down and participate in a demonstration project in which they would collaborate in building a LEGO set using the Engineer, Builder, and Parts-Supplier division of labor. Baron Cohen was one of the first to put up his hand to participate, so he sat with two other adults and collaborated on building a LEGO set. Later, we talked about that experience, and he said there might be something to this idea: it felt like something a child with autism would want to do. The LEGO building process offers a structure that is part of the overall system which guides not only the building project but the interpersonal interaction and communication process as well. You do not need to worry about what you are going to say or how you are going to interact with the other group members: the task demands make those obvious. Sir Simon later asked if he could have one of his graduate students from Cambridge visit with me in New Jersey to observe the groups I was running there and try to learn how to set up and run LEGO Club groups. He said the method seemed to capitalize on the children's natural systematic reasoning abilities to help with their social learning and social problem solving.

Baron Cohen's experience of collaborative LEGO building was not unlike that of many of the first children who participated in the groups in my playroom in Honolulu. Of course, at that time, the increase in the incidence and prevalence of autism was just getting started, and there were few pediatric developmental specialists in Hawaii at the time who were knowledgeable or experienced enough to take on a leadership role in developing educational and therapy programming for them. As a result, my child psychology and neuropsychology practice became increasingly focused on this population (I continued to work with children with a variety of issues, but mostly with neuro-developmental or neurocognitive disabilities). The transition from a couple of children interested in LEGO to a handful happened in a matter of weeks, and then from a handful of children to dozens of children happened in a few months.

The playroom was quickly almost entirely taken over by LEGO, and I became one of their best customers (I was paying and to this day I still pay retail for LEGO materials, and I have no direct affiliation with LEGO Corporation). Regarding the cost of other private practice materials like cognitive testing equipment and waiting room furniture, this was not a big deal, but it did provide me with a wonderful opportunity to create a sense of culture and community. The first few children who participated in LEGO Club began to show improvements in social interaction and communication that surprised everyone, including their teachers, parents, and siblings. They insisted on coming to LEGO Club on time every week, if not early, and they talked about LEGO Club when they were not there. We never referred to LEGO Club as LEGO therapy, or as a social skills group; it was always just the LEGO Club. Other children in the public school system heard about it from the participants and wanted to join. They thought it was just a private LEGO Club, like Boy Scouts or a community baseball team. The children's siblings wanted to join, and parents—including fathers for the first time—were so curious about what was happening they wanted to come in and watch.

Like most decisions in LEGO Club, I wanted to make sure that the group members felt this was their group, not mine, or their parents, so we were democratic about who should be allowed in. Parents were not allowed. Although the first few group members were boys, it wasn't long before we had a girl in the group, and then girls in the groups, and that worked surprisingly well. The girls were creative builders and that was all anyone cared about in that setting. They quickly became part of the ongoing system, but also added to the diversity of the group, having unique and un-boy-like ideas about what could be achieved using LEGO, including creations that were primarily esthetic, and did not have laser blasters, jet engines, or machine guns. The groups were divided along developmental lines, and over time there were enough children active in the groups, or on a waiting list for the groups, that we were able to assign them based on being closer in age, developmental level, and even temperament.

Some of the more frequent questions I am asked about LEGO Club have to do with the makeup of the groups. What many other professionals were surprised about was how easily autistic children who had minimal language proficiency could participate alongside children with exceptional language abilities. This was often due to the reciprocal nature of the LEGO Club collaborative synergy. Many children with limited language abilities have advanced visual-spatial and visual-motor abilities, while many children with overdeveloped vocabularies and adult-like syntax have more limited fine and gross motor skills and are not as skilled with complex LEGO construction tasks. In the context of LEGO Club, where the language of choice was LEGO, the children hardly noticed whether a peer was engaging in erudite banter or echolalia: they were too busy building.

With the growth of the groups from three or four to five or six and then seven to nine group members, it was necessary to add some skilled helpers. In general, the adult to child ratio was generally one to three for the younger groups (preschool to middle childhood), and then one for every five or six children for the older children (late elementary, middle school and up). Many of the groups of older children (ten years and older) required hardly any input or supervision except in exceptional circumstances, like someone bringing food into the LEGO room, or inviting their siblings or cousins, or friends from school. The therapists in LBT were able to focus almost entirely on coaching the social interaction and social communication because most of the children already knew how to participate with the LEGO materials themselves. Participating in LBT was not about learning to play with LEGO; it was about learning to play with other children. What emerged from that experience, however, was what was therapeutic: contributing to and benefiting from a sociocultural system and experiencing both the synergistic outcome of the group—efficient LEGO creativity that would have been out of reach of any individual group member—and of the group members—sharing a sense of value for the club and for each other.

Many of the children who were referred to my practice at that time were attending public and private schools, and the participants' attendance in the groups was funded by either their school district's special education division, or their parents' health insurance. There were also some children who attended private special needs schools, and at a couple of those schools, LEGO Club groups were set up and were able to operate on site during the lunch break or as an after-school activity. Some public schools also had more than a few children of similar ages who had autism and did not have a social development group, so a few groups were set up in public schools as well. At that time, I was the only person leading the groups, and I had some graduate students and post-doctoral supervisees attend groups with me as co-therapists. For many of them, there was a steep learning curve to catch up to some of the participants' proficiency with LEGO, but as we soon found out, that was not a necessity. The participants in LEGO Club were inevitably happy to demonstrate their skills and knowledge about LEGO by coaching a young adult therapist.

While the initial groups were focused on collaborative LEGO set-building, the members were also interested in doing freestyle creating, which is a much more demanding and complex process. Of course, many children can just put LEGO bricks together without following a set of directions, but that is not what was called for in LEGO Club. For group members to engage in freestyle building, they had to follow the cardinal rule of LEGO Club, which was to work on projects together. That meant they had to be able to communicate an idea for a freestyle to the other group members and do so in a way that convinced them to collaborate or share their skills, time, and energy on someone else's project. This requirement to collaborate on projects was always a catalyst for productive problem-generating and problem-solving. Even the set building was often problematic because the group members would have to agree about getting a new set, and then how they were going to assemble it—who was doing what, when, and for how long. Sometimes an entire group session would be taken up with disagreements and bartering of favors and promises regarding what set they should have me buy next. The magazines and catalogues would be out on the tables, and the participants would be shouting, gesturing, and demanding each other's and my attention and interest.

At the time I was not sure if this was going to be productive or not. In hindsight, I realize that it was probably the best possible form of therapy, but at the time the parents and the participants seemed to be quite unhappy with me if I let the bickering with each other go on and no LEGO sets got built. For a while I tried out a token economy system, which was introduced to objectively trade favors and keep track of them. I made a lot of LEGO tokens (small red squares of laminated paper with "LEGO" on them) which I offered to the participants quite generously at first for any prosocial, cooperative, and helpful actions. I offered them the opportunity to trade in the points they earned for a small or medium-sized LEGO set. I also allowed them to trade the LEGO points to each other to get other group members to support their choice of the project for the day, or to help them with a building project.

For a while, the group member who had the most LEGO points at the beginning of the group would inevitably get to lead the group, and some group members were savvy about using that to their advantage to require group members to give them even more points for them to participate in favorite roles in the construction process. In other words, the LEGO point system turned into an inflationary economy quickly. Somewhat surprising to me, though, was that the group members were much more interested in using their LEGO points to influence each other than they were in acquiring the new LEGO sets I had offered them. For a while, the group members dutifully kept track of all the red pieces of laminated paper, but after a few weeks, the tokens seemed like a hindrance. Like paper money, after a while it just disappeared from the economic exchanges: they became adept at keeping track of who owed whom, and they called in favors based on a new set of values, which reflected not just the jobs they did for each other, and the privilege of choosing the activity, or being in charge, but the value they showed for each other's unique and creative talents.

In addition to the growing scale of freestyle projects—which were done the younger groups based on rough sketches, and in the older groups involved elaborate blueprints and lengthy materials lists—in the later 1990's when there were about ten LEGO Club groups per week in my private office in the evenings and weekends, and another six or more in schools during the day. The participants' parents began to have informal gatherings amongst themselves. They met in the waiting room and often engaged in impromptu meetings or parent support groups in the parking lot outside my office. Teachers and special education therapists in the school system came to some of the groups with me to be "trained," in this new method. The fact that LBT was being offered by the school district on the island of Oahu became an issue in the state legislature because groups were not being offered on other islands. A graduate student from Maui began attending groups in my office on weekends so that he could bring the LEGO Club to the school system on that island.

During this time, some of the older group members also began to make scenes using LEGO and they painted backdrops and then took still photos of the scenes, which we had printed and blown up. Over time there was a growing collection of LEGO posters, and then photos of participants and their LEGO collections at home, or their creations with their friends in LEGO Club, including many of these scenes. By that time, LEGO had introduced the Star Wars collection, and other film-themed sets, so the LEGO scenes took on a cinematographic flair. Then a group member introduced the idea of using a LEGO scene to do a stop motion animated film. In fact, it was one of the first group members, Sam, who wanted to do a version of the Apollo 13 story using the LEGO space explorer's collection in a stop-motion format. At that time, shooting and editing stop-motion animation was a very clumsy process—the stop motion itself has not changed, but today children can accomplish what took us hours with VHS or Super-8 film in minutes using an app on a mobile phone, tablet, or laptop computer. Despite the tedious process, the result was striking, and the group members enjoyed helping on the project, and then sharing it with the other groups.

From early on, the multiple groups that were running during the week in the LEGO room were aware of each other's projects, of course, and were often competitive with each other. A few times this turned into formalized competitions such as building a tower of bricks from the tabletop to the ceiling of the LEGO room, or trying to build a stadium that would hold hundreds of mini-figs. Children's parents even started contributing ideas and funds to purchase LEGO for their group, like fund-raising for a baseball or soccer team, and buying them better uniforms or equipment. Some parents even contributed whole collections of new LEGO sets to the group. Of course, the advent of the first stop-motion animated short film was a clear challenge to all the other groups: Make a LEGO movie.

At about the time that LEGO stop-motion animation was getting started, my family and I had made the decision to relocate from Hawaii closer to family in New Jersey. I kept in touch with the original LEGO families and wrote about many of them in my second book, but unfortunately, those groups did not continue as I had hoped they might. In New Jersey, it took a while to convince anyone at my new employment setting, Bancroft Neurohealth, that a LEGO Club was a form of therapy and not just an obsession of mine. In the transition from Hawaii to New Jersey, though, I had found some spare that allowed me to go through the many files and reports that I had collected during my years in Hawaii, and I was able to put together a retrospective outcome study (LeGoff, 2004). As a result of both putting together that first study, and then just boldly taking over an underutilized conference room and filling it with LEGO, Bancroft's administration agreed to let me start a LEGO Club group. Among the die-hard behavior analysts who were well established at Bancroft as one of the premiere ABA services organizations, LEGO Club was still considered a rather silly experiment, but even the toughest-nosed behavior analysts were still curious enough to peer in to see what all the excitement was about.

The reception for the LEGO Club in the community in Cherry Hill and surrounding area—both privately and in the public school system—was just as spontaneous and immediate as it had been in Hawaii. Of course, in New Jersey there was considerably more competition and there were many active and reportedly successful social skills groups active and thriving. Jed Baker's Social Skills Training Project was being run just up the road in Springfield, New Jersey, and there were literally hundreds of autism ABA consultants offering social development programs for autistic children all over the state, not to mention just across the bridge in the Philadelphia area. Despite this, and without doing any kind of marketing or advertising, the word about a LEGO Club for autistic children began to spread, and referrals trickled in, and then poured in. It was around that time that I met Baron Cohen for the first time, and he convinced a doctoral student, Gina Owens (later, Gina Gomez de la Cuesta) to visit me in New Jersey outside Philadelphia and learn about LEGO Clubs.

It was Gina's idea to try to replicate the LEGO Club model using undergraduate students as therapists at Cambridge University and compare the LEGO Club model to that of an established social development therapy, the Social Use of Language Programme (SULP; Owens, *et al*, 2008). For her to do that, she needed to have a training manual for LBT, which did not exist at the time, except as a loose bunch of ideas in my head. The LEGO Club was not yet LBT, even though we had over time established some rules. Although the group members had given up on the LEGO points idea, one of the traditions of LEGO Club groups was the use of proscriptive rules, which were usually developed by the group members themselves, and which were typically posted in the LEGO room. The groups had also begun to benefit from using an informal set of social rules or norms which were not written and posted but which the group members began to understand and use in the groups and in other settings, and which I had dubbed, "The Rules of Cool," which are discussed below.

To assist Gina with her dissertation work, I agreed to have her attend several LEGO Club groups with me. I also wrote what seemed to me to be the emerging structure and system of the LBT process. In addition to Gina, there were two post-doctoral fellows, Sarah Levin, and GW Krauss, who were also participating in the groups, and they later helped provide some coherence and structure to what a very organic process had been. None of those who were involved, though, felt optimistic about the idea. LEGO Club just did not seem like something that could be manualized. At the same time, we agreed that we were not going to be able to share this idea without allowing an independent replication study and that required being able to communicate the method to naïve therapists who were themselves not personally invested in it as a method. My own perspective was that LEGO Club seemed to be the most expensive and inefficient group therapy imaginable, but there was something almost magical about the effect a roomful of LEGO had on a group of kids with autism: They just belonged there together, and they knew it.

Despite our misgivings about what could happen to LEGO Club if we offered it up, the LBT manual was handed off to Gina and her supervisors at Cambridge, including Sir Simon. That venture was later published as the first independent outcome study on LBT (Owens, *et al*, 2008). In the meantime, I had been able to get together with another colleague, the clinical and school psychologist, Michael Sherman, to generate another outcome study (LeGoff & Sherman, 2006). This was a longer-term study (three-year follow-up), which was also based on data that was collected in Hawaii. A couple of years after that was published, Gina and her colleagues gathered the data from their control-group study. That replication study was well received internationally, and more attention began to be paid to the idea of using LEGO as a play material for group therapy with autistic children. That spark ignited an international movement that has continued to today, with groups based on the LBT manual running in over fifty countries, with the highest concentrations of them in the UK, which were offshoots of Gina's initial replication groups at Cambridge.

LEGO Club as a Sociocultural System. In my informal relationship with the group members, they often seemed to accept my input, partly because they knew it was me (and my magic credit card) that paid for the LEGO. They also sensed that I meant well and was sincerely trying to be helpful when I would give a *sotto voce* tip, "That's not cool. Try something else." I would give hints to the group sometimes if a proscriptive or rule of cool was being broken and invite the group members—especially the more senior members—an opportunity to identify for the group that something was happening that was not acceptable, or not cool. "Cool," was a code word for "acceptable," "appropriate," or "helpful," but we generally emphasized that it contributed to the synergy of the group. Participating creatively in the synergistic process of the group was *cool*. That was also the *how* and *why* of collaborating with your friends: how you acted was cool or not, and why you acted that way was to be cool or not. Sometimes we had to back up and figure out where strong emotions like resentment or jealousy, feeling left out, or feeling stressed out and under pressure came from, since those feelings could result in any of us acting in ways that were not cool. Talking about how we made each other feel sometimes, or how the way someone acted interfered with what the group wanted to achieve, invariably led back to the topic of the unspoken, unwritten rules of cool.

After many years of running LEGO Club groups, many of the parents showed an interest in learning more about what was happening in the groups. Many of the children would share with their parents about the experiences they had in the group, but to maintain the sense of boundary around the Club, only group members were allowed to attend, not parents, or siblings, or personal friends. We did occasionally have visitors to the group, but they were always identified being part of the "therapist," or "teacher," category, who were part of my life experience, not theirs. From the group members' perspective, the group represented a synergistic system which was an extension of their self-system; it was important to them, valued by them, and it became integrated into how they experienced themselves and the systems around them. The families involved supported and participated in aspects of the LEGO Club, but they were not in the inner circle of it. Most of the participants intuitively understood that the power of the group for them was to some extent dependent on the Club being separated from other systems, outside influences, and outside events.

Just like all adaptive, synergistic systems, the LEGO Club had a semi-permeable boundary, which included having visitors (mostly other therapists and trainees), and life events that originated *out there*. Those experiences included experiences at home, school, and in community settings which were brought up as part of the discussion when they were relevant to the self-systems of the group members, and to the system of the group. It was important for the group members to consider the influence of life experiences since they had an impact on their actions in the group, directly and indirectly, but unlike *out there* where those experiences could be intense, stressful, frightening, and overwhelming, in the LEGO Club, which was a safe, calm, predictable, and fun place, we could share and talk about scary and confusing events, learn about them, understand them, and even overcome them.

One of the notable features of LEGO Club which I have described previously was the contribution made by parents separately from the Club, but in ways which allowed introduction of relevant outside influences through the appropriate channels, which was me as the therapist. In addition to the LEGO Club group, it was common for the participants to see me for individual and family therapy as well, and in those sessions, we focused on experiences and problems affecting the family, in school, and in the community. These were experiences that were clearly separate from what was happening in the LEGO Club, but there was a way for them to overlap when we used the *Rules of Cool* and other interpersonal coping strategies in both settings. If a child was experiencing a problem at home with parents or siblings, or with peers on the playground, or with a teacher in school, we could help the child apply a social norm or rule which applied to both that setting and LEGO Club.

In individual and family therapy sessions, children would take the opportunity to complain about, or actively engage in, a conflict or problem which originated at home, on the playground, or in the LEGO Club, but now directly with me. In adult psychotherapy, this is referred to as *transference*, which is the introduction of problematic experiences in the therapeutic relationship. A child who has been teased or bullied at school, or who feels unfairly treated at home, will necessarily react to those experiences in those settings, but most of the time their actions are not successful in resolving the problem. From the point of view of the model developed in this book, the child's self-system does not have an internal representation of the degrees of freedom of interpersonal systems which allow them to predict and to adaptively participate in those systems. To use a sports analogy again, this would be like a child experiencing a problem on the soccer field, the basketball or tennis court, which is frustrating and limiting their participation. They have not been able to create a solution for the problem, because they do not have the necessary degrees of freedom of that system internalized. Therapy, in that analogy, is like getting individualized coaching or tutoring, and in those sessions working on child's knowledge and skills relevant to the game.

The *Rules of Cool* were not intended to be set of rules but represented the norms and expectations that were not being intuitively developed by the child since they were not typically identifying with others or paying attention to the typical patterns of interpersonal and group interaction and communication. Just the idea that being socially competent, or cool, might involve following a set of unspoken rules was often a breakthrough insight for them. As was discussed earlier in this book, insight and understanding are not always necessary for adaptive participation in a system, which can be accomplished through procedural skills or knowledge. All organisms adaptively participate in ecosystems without conscious insight into their roles and strategies in that system. Conscious insight and understanding are unique features of adaptive competence which give us humans with large frontal lobes the advantage of being able to be more flexible and creative about how we participate in systems, but insight is not strictly necessary.

It was known, or at least acknowledged, by the participants in LEGO Club that the process of collaborating on LEGO projects was *cool*. The children and the therapists knew that there was something more about LEGO Club than LEGO-building, just as the leadership at LEGO Corporation and the massive numbers of child and adult fans of LEGO around the world accept that LEGO is about more than putting plastic bricks together. They intuitively know that their individual contributions to a shared cultural experience is more than just an individual or group activity; it has the synergistic outcome of a cultural experience that results in identification with others and a sense of commitment or affiliation with them. That intuitive knowledge is what is so hard to describe about play because it is not part of the process itself, but a synergistic emergent outcome of it: play is a way of identifying with and creatively participating in culture.

Building LEGO is doubly synergistic because in addition to the individual activity creating the community and culture of LEGO fans, a LEGO builder is also making something more than the sum of the bricks themselves: it is a symbolic representation. In some cases, a child or adult will put bricks together in a non-representational way, which is perhaps even functional (I have business card holder on my desk made of LEGO bricks, and there are lots of ways to engineer functional objects out of LEGO bricks) but there is nothing special about those creations: they are not playful because they do not relate to culture. Culture reflects communication, technology, and interpersonal norms of a group of people who rely on that culture as an element of their adaptation.

The description of play activities as behaviors by ABA misses the emergent dimension of culture itself, which is the point: play is not something children do just to improve their cognitive development; it is also how they learn to be creative and share their creativity with others. The misunderstanding of language as verbal behavior, skills as learned behavior, or innovation as free operants grossly distort the constructivist and evolutionary models which identify these as integral components of emergent shared systems like language, technology, and social norms. Culture evolves and grows because individual humans play together and thereby share the emergent results with both each other and a growing, thriving culture (Burghardt, 2015; LaFreniere, 2011; van Schaik & Burkhart, 2011; Gaskins, Haight, & Lancy, 2006; Goncu, Jain, & Teurmer, 2006; van Schaik, Deaner, & Merrill, 1999).

According to Corning (2022), life forms, species, and ecosystems evolved through collaborative synergy. That same principle has also been used to explain human evolution and our adaptive use of cultural systems (Corning, 2018, 2011). That is a way of thinking about human interdependence that resonates with our intuitive understanding of how sociocultural systems work. Families, educational systems, and communities provide the stability that benefits us as individuals and those stable systems benefit from our diverse, creative input. This exchange allows for a balance of stability and flexibility which is the hallmark of adaptable organic systems (Corning, 2022; 2005; 2003; Drack, 2015; von Bertalanffy, 1968a & b).

The LEGO Club experience offers two synergistic experiences to children simultaneously: LEGO as a play material, and LEGO as a social group and shared culture. Many children have LEGO at home, but what most do not have is the experience of interpersonal synergy and shared creativity which comes from being in a LEGO Club. As Göncü and Gaskins (2006), have documented, social play is a central part of both human evolutionary history and social development in children. Without understanding the hierarchical systems involved in development and attempting to reduce it to cause-effect relationships between behavior, genes, or neurons, the representational nature of autism is missed. Autistic children operate perfectly fine as living organisms, the problem is not with their physiology or behavior, the problem is with their relationship to their sociocultural context.

Collaborative LEGO building is an intensely interpersonal experience. Even though children are necessarily focused on the instructions and the bricks, they are also required to focus on each other's hands, faces, and voices. Joining a LEGO Club group means being asked to keep up with a group of peers who may be even more adept at a skill you value than you are yourself. That can be challenging, but most children who are new to LEGO Club groups intuitively know that they are among friends, and that their presence and contributions are valued by the other group members. The projects are designed to require the contributions of all members, whether that is just sorting bricks in a tray or taking charge of an entire project. The two systems involved in LEGO Club, the sociocultural and the material, interface and influence each other, in complex ways, but in general there is also a synergistic dynamic between them. Just building LEGO or just being part of a social skills group do not have the impact on social and communication of the interaction of these experiences. While this synergistic interaction effect has its effects on participants in intuitive, unconscious ways, the group also offers some explicit ways to represent this developmental progress: the *Rules of Cool*, and the *Level System*.

The *Rules of Cool*, as mentioned above, were not intended to be like the LEGO Club Rules, which were written proscriptive rules, but these were often part of the conversations the group members had about the interpersonal issues in the room, and often came up in conversations about outside issues. These were often introduced to the group by the therapists, including me, who would know that certain group members were struggling with certain issues and that they might need some practice with a certain interpersonal skill or to have input from their valued peers about how they were dealing with similar issues in their lives. Quite often the group members would refer to the *Rules of Cool* that they understood and used as social norms, and which helped them to solve problems or proactively avoid them. The younger, less well-developed children learned to use simpler, less nuanced versions of *Rules of Cool* that were appropriate for their peer interactions.

Rules, Roles, and Levels in LEGO Club. If it was not made clear earlier, it should be emphasized that the LEGO Club and its designation, LEGO-based therapy (LBT), in outcome studies are the result of an organic process. By that I mean that there was no initial theoretical rationale or ideological structure towards which it was directed. The Club itself was formed at the initiation of the children. Having a LEGO Club was not my idea, or something that the children's parents asked for; it was formed because autistic children wanted to get together and build LEGO. They thought that would be fun, and so their parents and I facilitated that. The next thing that happened was my idea, the requirement to build interactively and collaboratively, but that was based on my prediction that they might otherwise engage in parallel activities, and not interact directly. It was a bit surprising to me then, and it is still surprising to many professionals who try this method, that the children are accepting of this arrangement.

It is inevitable that there will be children in LEGO Club groups who struggle with the expectation for them to collaborate with others, but those children are often not in the group because they are autistic. It is more common for this situation to arise in the context of children who have another condition, such as ADHD, ODD, or some other externalizing factors (disruptive, aggressive, narcissistic conditions), or a co-morbid combination of autism or BAP and then psychological reactance or disinhibition of affect. In my experience, children who present with an uncomplicated BAP or autism are not opposed to social collaboration, they are just not good at it. Being poor at a skill-based activity naturally results in a decreased level of motivation for that activity, as has been discussed at length in this book. It is understandable then that a child whose self-system—and the conscious component of that self-system, their self-image—does not include an adequate sub-system of interpersonal guidelines which allows them to creatively participate in peer-group activities is not going to be eager to initiate that sort of activity.

One of the most frequent questions I receive from providers who attend LBT training is about dealing with oppositional, disruptive, and aggressive tendencies in the group members. These are not the result of being autistic. If a child was born with low sociality or the BAP and has subsequently experienced events which resulted in maladaptive patterns of interpersonal coping that include reactance and low stress tolerance, that will be noticeable immediately when we introduce them to the idea of collaborative LEGO-building. That is why I recommend spending some time with a child one-on-one with LEGO materials—including set-building and some freestyle creating (LeGoff, et al, 2014)—to build a sense of trust and alliance with them, and to get them accustomed to the basic component activities: finding the right bricks, following a plan, and putting bricks together. Introducing them to a group before they have acquired some proficiency with those basic skills may require them to learn those skills on the fly in the group, but that is not impossible, and many group members will be happy to help them. If the problem is not the LEGO skills, but that the child is just not interested in the activity without being disruptive and oppositional, that is not the same problem.

The group members will often want to introduce others to their proscriptive rules, like using an indoor voice, not climbing on furniture, or putting things back where they belong, but that is often a form of indoctrination into the group membership, more than a necessary boundary-setting. More important to them, they will want to introduce a group member to the LEGO building process—what they need to do to collaborate with the other group members in their activities—and then soon they (and the therapists) will be gently reminding them or modeling for them the *Rules of Cool*, which are social norms; the unspoken and invisible variables which regulate social competence. At some point, many of the participants would develop some insight about the interaction between being competent at the LEGO activities and being socially competent, and in fact, as is evident in the Level System described below, it was an explicit goal of the group members to become competent at both. Eventually the participants' parents became curious to know more about the *Rules of Cool*, and the *Level System*, which were both just organic emergences of the group's ongoing homeostatic operations. The LEGO Club started out with distinct roles, which were required to initiate collaborative building and shared creativity, but it did not start out with rules and levels. For the group to persist and to grow and replicate itself, like any synergistic, adaptable system, it needed some stability and structure, and those just evolved naturally out of the collaborative efforts of the group members, with some input from the leaders.

The need to formally describe the *Rules of Cool* and the *Level System* in some written form resulted initially from the participants talking to their parents about their participation in the group. Not all parents, but some of them who may not have had an intuitive understanding of why the LEGO Club had social rules (norms), or a hierarchy based on accomplishments, did ask for some objective description of these guiding principles and benchmarks. Despite my hesitancy about putting something that should be flexible and adaptable in writing, I did offer some parents a written form of the *Rules of Cool*. For the younger participants, and those who were learning the basics of interpersonal competence, I described the kinds of skills and the focus that the therapists had in those groups in terms of what we might be prompting and supporting the group members to practice and improve on, which were labelled, "Easy Rules of Cool." For the older children and those who already had achieved the basic level of interpersonal competence, I wrote out a set of "Serious Rules of Cool."

I did not share these documents with the participants, though, since that would have been distracting and possibly have led to the sort of rigid and *pro forma* sort of compliance that I had seen in other sorts of social skills groups which had a behavioral focus. What was happening in the LEGO Club remained natural (not "naturalistic"), child-led, organic, and synergistic, including the children learning together how to be friendly, helpful, supportive, polite, calm, generous, and conscientious, or in other words, how to be cool.

Easy Rules of Cool

1. I like people, so I look at them and smile.
2. I like to make a good impression, so I get clean and dress carefully.
3. I don't want to scare anyone, so I move my hands slow and low.
4. If I'm not sure what to do, I get a little help from my friends.
5. Unless I'm invited in, I stay out of people's personal space.
6. I don't touch anyone, or let them touch me, unless I know them very well.

Serious Rules of Cool

1. I like people, so when I look at them, I smile.
2. I don't worry about small stuff; if something minor bothers me, the best thing to do is forget about it and move on.
3. I listen to people and think about what they are saying before I respond.
4. I make myself heard, but I'm never louder than I need to be.
5. I think about what I wear so I fit in, but I know clothes are just the surface.
6. If I have something good to say, I offer to share; otherwise, I listen.
7. I get ready for the day early so I'm not late, or in a rush.
8. I give people their space: stand a few feet away, and don't ask personal questions.
9. I notice when someone is busy, and I don't bother them; I wait.
10. I don't repeat myself or talk too long about the same thing.

Having communicated these "rules," to parents and others, who were never intended as rules, I do not recommend coming up with a set of rules and then using them as a set of prompts or behavioral goals. They are intended to represent the typical sorts of social norms that many autistic children miss or do not learn because they have not been participating in interpersonal systems throughout their development. What the therapists in LEGO Club are typically doing is prompting the participants to pay attention to how they are interacting with each other in ways that sometimes leads to conflicts or misunderstandings, or which interfere with their experience of identification and affiliation with each other. This is not following rules but noticing and internalizing the variables that are relevant to adaptively participating in a sociocultural system. Just as importantly, rules tend to be limiting, and should be viewed instead as principles or values to aspire to, but "Principles of Cool," or "Aspirational Values of Cool," just did not sound right.

The LEGO Club *Level System* was also an outgrowth of the participants' LEGO activities and their relationships with each other and the group, and it shows even more clearly how the LEGO Club was able to combine the synergistic systems of LEGO play materials with the Club as an organization. As was described earlier and in previous writing about LEGO Club, the division of labor (Builder, Parts-Supplier, and Engineer) was initially an attempt on my part to ensure that the participants would engage in joint attention, interpersonal communication, and collaboration with joint accomplishment. As the group evolved, however, the activities changed and so the roles also changed. At first, the transition to freestyle building meant that there needed to be a designer, like an architect, who came up with the overall idea and physical outline of what they wanted to build, but they still might need some help with the engineering of that model. That naturally meant that the roles were no longer on one level and could be interchanged as we had been doing with the *triad model* and set building, switching roles periodically.

The *Level System* was a necessary adaptation in the group once the group had been running for a while and new members began to join. Some of the new group members had well-developed LEGO skills, but they were not necessarily proficient in following the LEGO Club procedures, and there was some need among the group members to identify the competency of group members both in terms of their LEGO skillset and their interpersonal skillset. The group members experienced for themselves that sometimes a new group member would want to jump right into designing a freestyle creation, but they had not earned any credit with the other group members to get them to do the hard building work for them, they also had not earned the other group member's respect as having the LEGO skills needed to come up with a buildable design (like a novice architect handing over unworkable designs to experienced engineers). Finally, the new group members had not developed the interpersonal skills to be able to communicate about and organize the tasks relevant to their ideas. A new group member had to first demonstrate to the other participants that they could build, design, communicate, and manage the group dynamics before they could plunge into having the group take on a project for them.

The first division of levels was instituted by the original group members when some additional participants joined the group later. They wanted to make sure that a new group member could competently participate in the three basic roles of Engineer, Parts-supplier, and Builder, as well as being able to independently complete other basic tasks which were part of the freestyle building process like sorting parts, finding a part as described by another group members, doing pre-assembly, or disassembly and then sorting pieces into the correct storage bins. The more experienced participants would identify a new group member as a *helper* until such a time that they felt they had demonstrated to them that they were competent as a *builder*. Then, there were builders who were adept at putting sets together or helping on freestyle builds who were still learning how to design or engineer freestyle creations. This was a problem if they were allowed to lead a group activity, and the other group members were then trying to work on a set that was difficult or impossible to construct.

Among the group members, there was recognition for the LEGO Corporation's series Creator Sets, which often had the option of being able to modify and customize them, and so they began to refer to group members who were adept at freestyle designing as Creators. That naturally led to what became the next level after Helper and Builder. The sorts of LEGO creations that could be envisioned and implemented by LEGO Creators varied considerably in size and complexity, as well as in overall esthetic appeal. The group members tried out a variety of ways to evaluate the quality of freestyle creations, such as the frightening "drop test," which involved purposely dropping a LEGO design from about tabletop height to assess a design's engineering integrity (the more pieces that flew off, the worse the design rating). There were many other variables of course, such as face validity (you could tell what it was supposed to be), esthetic appeal (color scheme and shape), size, complexity, and even how well it dovetailed with other creations (did it fit into the collection?), adding novelty as well as continuity.

At some point the terms "Expert Builder," and then "Expert Creator," began to be used in reference to the most experienced and accomplished group members who had been successful in leading the group on the completion of a complex group project, especially ones which required schematics, sometimes prototypes, and then materials lists, and the assignment of tasks, including sub-groups who might be working on a part of the project, or doing some prep work with sorting, collecting bricks, and pre-assembly. A group member who could take a leadership role like a project manager on a multi-session creation would need to accept feedback and criticism, as well as communicate accurately and carefully with group members, while maintaining their motivation and commitment to the project. Many successful Creators, who had excellent design ideas and knew how to engineer innovative and creative projects, failed at the group leadership process by being impatient, changing their directions or priorities, not allocating adequate time, and then putting everyone under too much pressure, or just losing control of their emotions when there were problems instead of using the group as a resource.

Later, a Creator for whom it was important to be recognized by the group as a "Master" wanted to be formally recognized. This was somewhat of an issue at times when the group would discuss each other's contributions and skills and some members felt slighted or not fully recognized or valued for their contributions. It also became somewhat of a contentious status issue, and even a chain-of-command problem during complex projects that some-one in charge would offer a task to a Helper, when a LEGO Builder or Creator may have been available to do the job. The group members took these sorts of decisions seriously because they knew that if they helped with an import-ant job on a big build, when it came time for them to try to get their idea accepted, or to get other skilled members to help them with the project, they would need to use that credit to influence them.

Group members at the LEGO Master level were showing considerable social competence, motivation, and even self-confidence and assertiveness outside of the group setting. This was invariably aided by the participant hav-ing been in the group for a while, and their parents and other family members having a relationship with other group members, so they had experiences out-side of the Club, but related to the Club: LEGO Club birthday parties, grad-uations, bar mitzvahs and bat mitzvahs, Fourth of July, and Christmas parties, etc. The typical pattern for most group members who moved up through the levels so that they were competent enough with both LEGO and the socio-cultural systems involved was that they often became involved in other social activities outside the Club, such as being able to be on a sports team, joining another club, a choir, or a youth band or orchestra, succeeding in Boy or Girl Scouts of America, or just having a lot of friends and playdates.

Note: The term, "Master," can have associations and connotations of social injustice and slavery. While this term, as used by the children in LEGO Club, was never intended to convey more than having mastered the art and skill of creating with LEGO materials, it would be insensitive and potentially hurtful not to acknowledge that for some children, families, cultures, and ethnic groups, the term *master* connotes mastery over others and not simply mastery of a skill or knowledge. Since there are synonyms available, such as the term *expert*, going forward in this manuscript and in future publications, the term Expert will be used in place of Master. I also encourage other LBT participants and therapists to consider using the term *LEGO Expert* in place of *LEGO Master*.

The result of the expanded outcome of social competence in group members was that their attendance declined or ended, or the parents and their IEP team, or their pediatrician or psychiatrist, or some combination of these would come to the decision that LEGO Club was no longer necessary. Quite often, well before that point, the participant and their parents and I would have been discussing the transition process. Ending involvement with the LEGO Club was sometimes not an issue since some group members had developed enough insight about the process that they understood that it was a social skills group for autistic children, and they no longer needed it, and were even sometimes a bit embarrassed by coming to groups. This happened especially when senior group members had not been to a group for a while, and then attended and got to meet some new group members who were clearly just learning how to work with LEGO, and to participate in an interpersonal system.

Many group members expressed their desire to return to the Club and continue to contribute, but it was not expected that this would be billed as group therapy. These group members were offered the opportunity to attend groups—their original group or other groups that occurred in that setting during the week—as volunteer mentors. The advent of peer mentors in the groups was a positive and synergistic one for both the groups and for those participants. The younger group members were able to identify with and model both the LEGO-based skillset and their interpersonal interaction and communication skills. For the LEGO Club graduates, this was also a positive sense of identity for them, since they were able to experience giving back to a sociocultural system which had benefitted them, and to have the experience of being an accomplished role model. Amongst the LEGO Club staff, parents, and participants, these graduates became identified as the LEGO Legends. This term was applied by one admiring young group member who met one of the graduates who had started that group, and there were photos of him and his creations on the walls in the group, and his name was on both large LEGO sets and photographs of LEGO creations on the wall. When the senior member was introduced as having once been a member of that group, the young group member said he already knew who he was, "You're a LEGO legend!"

Being a LEGO Legend was a big accomplishment, and well-deserved, as some members participated in the LEGO Club for years to reach that level. Other group members went through the levels much more quickly and were able to get what they needed from the groups, and quickly move on or fade out of their groups as their own lives became fuller and busier with socio-cultural activities. Many still enjoyed coming back to the groups on special occasions, like the anniversary of their first group, or the date of their graduation. Graduates and their families also tended to stay in touch with each other outside of the groups, and many are still friends today, decades after having been in the LEGO Club with each other.

A LEGO participant who had struggled valiantly for some time to achieve LEGO Master status, the other therapists and group members decided that we should recognize his achievement with a LEGO Master diploma. That became a popular idea, especially for group members who graduated, and we combined the giving of the LEGO level diploma with a graduation ceremony. The parents were delighted as much as anyone, and often brought cake, and some even had the diploma's framed and they brought pictures of the LEGO graduate's diploma on their wall at home. The LEGO Level certificate became an integral ritual of LEGO Club activities, and a key part of that was having the group members sign the diploma. The decision about a group member achieving a level was always left up to the other group members, but over time, the criteria for achieving each level became more formalized, and there were some objective ways for the group members to evaluate their achievement of the relevant skills and knowledge base. There was still room for debate about levels, especially at the higher levels, which led to some very productive discussions about how the group members valued each other's contributions, as well as the benefit-contribution balance of each member. Some talented members were acknowledged for their skills, but the other group members would not agree to advance them to the next level because they had been selfish and had not contributed in a balanced way to the other's projects.

When a new group member joined a LEGO Club, they had always been screened and prepared for the group by the lead therapist. The Club members had also been prepared for having a new group member attending, and the more senior group members would be asked to introduce themselves and the others, explain how the group operated, review the proscriptive rules, and the general idea that this was a Club and not a LEGO playroom, so collaborative participation was not optional. The new Helper would also have their roles identified and then they would be offered a role on an ongoing project—a set or a freestyle. The other group members also introduced themselves, or were introduced by more senior group members, and they might have their level described, for example: "This is Peter, he's still a Builder, but he's getting close to being a Creator. He's designing a gas station for Beth's town. Beth is almost a LEGO Master." Once the new participant had a chance to demonstrate their basic skills to the group, they might ask to move up a level, or the other group members might want them to step up to doing some freestyle building, and they would agree that it was time for them to get a LEGO Builder certificate.

For a while, the LEGO Master level was the highest level, and group members who graduated as Masters would recirculate as the LEGO Legends. After the advent of stop-motion animated filming, however, there was an even stronger motivation for participants to remain active. The stop-motion animation activity greatly increased the number of roles and the skill domains in addition to LEGO-based ones and the core social competencies. The main skill domain that was added by the stop-motion animation projects was shared creativity. In addition to creativity, of course there were other systems of knowledge and skill which were not part of either set building or freestyle creating, but the main challenge for most of the group members who were usually at the Creator or Master level in the groups was communicating about creative ideas, and then being able to collaborate in their execution.

The Emergence of LEGO Stop-Motion Films as a Group Activity. While being a project manager and having the social communication and assertiveness skills were required to achieve the LEGO Master level, over-seeing a stop-motion animation project using LEGO required many additional skills and offered many more challenges including task assignment and oversight of sub-groups which had their own internal hierarchies, time-management, and careful analysis of other group member's skills and aptitudes. A LEGO Club member who had an innovative idea for a LEGO-based stop motion film would need to sell that idea to their collaborators, banking on their established reputation for having the requisite skills, and the goodwill in the room. They would need to communicate the idea using a storyboard, or by borrowing a story from the media (typically a scene from a popular movie, or a recent sporting or other news event). They would also have to decide who should be responsible for which parts of the production process, often assigning more than one role to each member, getting Club members to audition for parts as voice-actors or animators, and being knowledgeable about their other skills, such as set-building, freestyle creating, and group leadership.

A successful stop-motion animation project required a wide range of roles and skillsets, and the member vying to get the Club's agreement to take on a project would be committing all of them to this project for several therapy sessions, as well as taking up possibly a considerable amount of space and materials in the room. The roles involved often included:

- Producer (usually the leader of project)
- Director (sometimes also the producer)
- Script writer
- Story-boarder
- Cinematographer
- Film, sound, and special effects editing
- Stop motion animators
- Voice-over actors
- Set designers
- Set builders
- Cue-card holders

During a project, the leader—the producer or director—would have to oversee a few parallel group activities over a series of sessions, sometimes interrupted by other group activities. The project could take months to complete, and in the process the plot and script might need to be revised, the sets and actors might be changed, group members who had roles as voice actors might graduate, or just not show up, etc. There were always complications involved, even when trying to shoot just a couple of minutes or less of an animated film. The technology involved changed dramatically over the time that stop-motion brick films were produced, and each new piece of film would be viewed by other groups and any innovations or creativity would be copied and replicated.

Some group members came up with stop motion filming ideas that were so compelling and effective that the other group members wanted to replicate and serialize them. Although many ideas were just LEGO-based knockoffs, using the readily available LEGO Star Wars, Spiderman, Batman, Harry Potter, Thomas the Tank Engine, and Sponge Bob Square Pants series. In addition to just replicating favorite scenes, the Club members also created satirical versions, and then whole new story lines or cross-over stories (e.g., Sponge Bob meets Spiderman). Quite a few group members, though, had creative ideas that were not innovative or derivative, such as a series called "Cindy Brickberg," which was an ill-fated on-the-scenes new anchor, or "Stuntman Biff," who was a comically clumsy and unambitious film stunt actor. There were many opportunities for the Club members to express off-color or politically incorrect themes or to satirize popular media in ways that were not always popular with their parents, or appropriate for their younger siblings, but they were very much grist for the mill of early adolescent sociocultural development.

The themes of the stop-motion films could be farcical or satirical—like the popular TV game show series, "Try Not to Die!"—but they also often explored sincere themes of social attachment, loyalty, anxiety, stress, or loss. The group members often spent time talking about the scripts and the message that was intended to be offered to a hypothetical audience. They understood that they were not just moving pieces to create the illusion of movement—although that was a skill, they all had to practice—but that they were trying to create a narrative which communicated about an experience which was intended to elicit emotions. It was therefore critical for them to have their stop-motion productions seen. At the end of many filming sessions, the group members would invite their parents, and anyone else who was in the waiting area, in for a screening of the day's rushes. Watching their own minute or two of stop-motion filming on a laptop screen, with their families present, was a special moment for all of them: the excitement and tension was palpable.

After years of sharing stop-motion animated shorts with each other and their families, the groups came up with the idea of having a LEGO film festival. This was partly due to the overlapping groups, who were intensely curious to see each other's productions and to compare notes on staging, special effects, voice acting, and sound editing. The groups would notice that another group was using a particular scene for their film, and would want to see the film, get ideas from it, and then want to borrow the idea, set, characters, and the whole lot. There was also just a general curiosity and interest in the other group members, which was like what I had observed in the original few children in my practice in Hawaii who were interested in the others whose LEGO creations they had seen on the bookshelves; they identified with each other and that lead to a motivation to affiliate. When the children met as a large group for the first LEGO film festival, hosted at the Center for

Neurological and Neurodevelopmental Health, the CNNH, in New Jersey, there were about seventy participants along with their parents, siblings, and other friends and relatives.

It turned out to be quite a large group. The group was so large, in fact, that we had to abandon having the large LEGO room and take over the lobby of the office complex we were in. We had edited more than an hour of short stop-motion animated films together, and we had the kids who had created them come up and introduced themselves. There were a few members of the press there in addition to the children and their families, so the LEGO Club participants got a taste of being celebrities at their own miniature version of Cannes or Sundance. Many of the LEGO Club members wanted to meet children from other groups whose work they admired and ask them questions about their ideas, technical skills, and their creative process. Many of the parents, siblings, and other family members were surprised by the size of the group and the enthusiasm for the amateur stop-motion productions. For many of them, it was the first time that they thought about their child has having abilities and talents that other children and adults understood and valued. Many of the friends and siblings who attended were envious of the obvious fun and technological achievement that was on display. On that day, LEGO Club truly was a valued sociocultural system, and a community.

Since then, with the publication of the LBT manual that was written initially for Gina Gomez de la Cuesta's doctoral thesis (Owens, *et al*, 2008), was published in English (LeGoff, *et al*, 2014), and then translated into multiple languages including Spanish, Italian, Portuguese, Polish, and Chinese. Gina and her colleague, Elinor Brett, who also did her doctoral thesis on LEGO therapy (Brett, 2013), have offered numerous training seminars on LBT in the UK and EU, and founded *Play Included*, which is now partnering with the *LEGO Foundation*—an international non-profit educational and child development organization. Gina and Elinor also collaborated with Barry Wright at the *Child Oriented Mental health Innovation Collaborative* (COMIC) at York University in the UK in completing a WHO-registered randomized controlled replication study on LBT at York, Hull, and Sheffield Universities. The project, *I-SOCIALISE*, used its own version of the LBT manual, and was one of the largest independent replication studies of LBT (Wright, *et al*, 2017).

Research on LEGO-Based Therapy. Following the initial two studies which were done by myself and my colleague, Michael Sherman, on generalized objective outcomes of LBT (LeGoff, 2004; LeGoff & Sherman, 2006), Gina and her colleagues at Cambridge University followed up with the first independent replication study, which compared LBT to the Social Use of Language Programme (SULP, Owens *et al*, 2008). Within a brief period, there were multiple independent replication studies (Levy & Dunsmuir, 2020; Nguyen, 2016; Yalamanchili, 2015; Evans, *et al*, 2014; Brett, 2013; Andras, 2012; Kato, Hatori, Iwai, & Morita 2012; Pang, 2010). Some of these studies utilized the LeGoff, *et al* (2014) LBT manual, but for the earlier studies, the method was communicated using the initial studies (LeGoff, 2004, LeGoff & Sherman, 2006, and Owens, *et al*, 2008), and then other informal training and supervision. These studies found consistent evidence that the basic idea of using a preferred play activity, LEGO building, as the basis for a social development group had a positive influence on social interaction and communication. Most of these studies used the first LBT manual, and the duration of treatment was typically much briefer than many of the LEGO Club groups that were run by me and colleagues directly. Nonetheless, the outcomes were promising, and many clinical researchers were interested in expanding the range of activities and including longer-term involvement and monitoring outcomes over longer periods of time.

Another set of studies were also published which focused on modifications or alternative applications of the original methodology described in the first outcome studies and the manual. The main form of modification was the use of school and classroom settings as opposed to outpatient clinics. While both of my first studies and then Owens, *et al* (2008) were done in clinic settings, several subsequent outcome studies were conducted in schools, and most of these were conducted by special education teachers and school psychologists, not clinical child psychologists. It should be noted that the Owens, *et al*, study utilized undergraduate psychology students as the primary therapists, but they were supervised by clinical psychologists. Evans and Bond (2021), followed Hu, Zheng & Lee (2018), Cheng (2016), MacCormack, *et al* (2015), and Boyne (2014) in using the LBT method for students identified with autism at school implemented by special education teaching staff, not child psychologists.

While the LEGO Club groups that we were running in outpatient clinics were showing generalized gains for children in their school settings—on the playground and at lunch breaks—as well as at home and in the community (based on the Vineland Adaptive Behavior Scales data), the integration of LBT into school settings was even more directly creating an interface between the LEGO system, LBT, and the children's own sociocultural environment. The goals and methods of clinic-based and school-based LBT did not differ significantly, but of course, there were some procedural and administrative issues which were different, including the fact that the school-based LBT was being provided as an educationally relevant intervention, and not as a mental health service.

In addition to the positive replication studies and generalization of LEGO Clubs from clinics to school settings, additional modifications of the method were recorded by occupational therapists and speech pathologists. These providers have slightly different goals and professional points of view from either child psychologists or educators, as well as often having somewhat different goals for group-based therapy with children diagnosed with autism. Kulju and Mäki (2017) are occupational therapists, based in Finland, who contacted me, and we collaborated on their use of the LeGoff *et al* (2014) manual as the basis for their trial of LBT as an occupational therapy group to improve both social interaction and fine motor and motor planning skills. Ralph and Rochester (2016) also contacted me about using LBT as the basis for group speech-language therapy sessions, and that collaboration led to their publication of their own therapy manual for speech pathologists.

Additional generalization studies have examined variations of the methodology using LEGO robotics activities (Barakova, *et al*, 2015), and this group also later combined robotics-mediated LEGO activities with sibling involvement (Huskens, *et al*, 2015). Both studies showed both immediate and longer-term gains, with sustained improvement in social communication and social competence with peers and siblings. The impact of LBT on social adjustment and communication with families was also assessed by Peckett, *et al* (2016), using parental interviews to collect data on the impact of LBT on family system functioning. Griffiths (2016), examined both parent and teacher observations and impressions of the effects of LBT on autistic children, finding that improvements in social competence at school were accompanied by positive changes with the family at home. Finally, there have been a few critical integrative reviews and meta-analytic studies of LBT reviewing the aggregate data and outcomes from the published original and replication studies (Narzisi, *et al*, 2021; Ramalho & Sarmento, 2019; Lindsay, *et al*, 2017; Strath, 2010).

Many of the replication, generalization, and review studies have commented on the strength of this intervention approach being its appeal to the participants: the children in LBT are typically eager to participate. The group process itself is also usually straightforward and both the therapists and participants have a clear sense of what they are supposed to be doing during LBT sessions. Based on feedback from other healthcare and mental health professionals who have visited LEGO Club sessions, and from those who have started and are running their own groups, the entire process has what they consider face validity, or what those in real estate would call 'curb appeal.' No one comes into a LBT session and wonders what is going on or why; the activity is visually apparent, the participants are enthusiastic, and focus of attention is a mutual creative activity. Although the waiting area can become a bit of a circus due to the excitement and anticipation, the LEGO Club is typically a serious place, with a lot of focused effort and technical communication. It is playful, but the sort of play that makes it clear that play is a learning process.

Disputes and disagreements, including heated exchanges, are also common in the room, but they have the quality of teammates disagreeing about a game strategy, or colleagues in the workplace vying to get credit for a successful project, or to shed blame for an unsuccessful one. Just like with teammates or co-workers, sometimes the relationships and emotions become more personal, and the LEGO Club members do have real relationships with each other, as do their families. That is a big part of what makes LEGO Club successful, though. It is playful, it is fun, and it is real to the participants. It is as real as a social setting as any classroom, playground, community, or home. That is one of the misconceptions that some adults have about play; just because children are playing does not mean the consequences are not real or important. Without play, there would be no culture, and without culture, there would be no human beings.

What the LEGO Club environment and the involvement of the adult therapists confirms for the participants is that they are valuable as members of society, and that what they want to do, what they are interested in, and what they create are important. Just as importantly, they identify with each other and they see how they and the other group members concur about what is valuable in their joint projects, as well as what is valuable about their actions towards each other. Identification and affiliation are the spark of recognition and desire to be with and to connect with our parents, which is a central organizing principle of life for most of us. For some of us, that experience is powerful, and we are born with an innate ability to observe and learn from other people all we need to know to creatively participate in sociocultural systems. People who are high on sociality are gregarious, charming, influential, the life of the party, or the group leaders.

Individuals who are high in traits of sociality are also vulnerable to problems that may arise from being overly dependent on others or have too much of their self-esteem and their coping abilities dependent on interpersonal acceptance and positive feedback. Most people are balanced in terms of being both self-reliant and able to benefit from and contribute to interpersonal and sociocultural systems. Other individuals who are low on sociality are not necessarily disabled or pathological in any way. It is just that in our current developmental and educational systems it is difficult for a child to get through the gauntlet of social systems without being labeled, especially if that child prefers to play in ways that are not social.

LEGO Club is a safe place, but it is also a realistically social environment. The good news for children with low sociality or autism is that there are other children just like you, and there are social coaches in the room to prompt you through the process. LEGO Club is the very definition of a user-friendly environment for autistic children. It is also the very definition of a synergistic system at both the interpersonal and material level. There are conscientiously developed levels to both which make it accessible for children at any level of LEGO building skill, and any level of interpersonal skill, so that each child's experience is that they can creatively contribute and benefit from the synergy in the room. They experience the value in both directions: each child is valued by the group, and the group is valuable to each child, and the outcome is developmental growth for both.

In the first LBT outcome study (LeGoff, 2004), after only a few months of weekly participation in a one-hour group therapy session, the participants increased the average amount of time they were interacting with peers on the playground at school by over 400%, from about 50 seconds total per recess break, to over four minutes. In the study, both self-initiated social contact and duration of social interaction during free play were recorded. Those values can be combined (number of interactions with duration of interactions) to calculate the total duration of social play. This may not seem like a huge change, but it is important to keep in mind the duration and frequency of therapy: once per week for an hour. LEGO-based therapy and the LEGO Club groups have continued to grow and increase in their range of creative activities, which enhances the experience for everyone involved.

CHAPTER 3

THE GOALS OF LEGO-BASED THERAPY

In what follows, there are many specific details about how LEGO Club groups have been established and run which may give the reader the impression that there is a single, preferred, and ideal method for doing LBT. That is not the main purpose of this book. The initial purpose for creating a manual for LBT (LeGoff, *et al*, 2014) was to facilitate an independent replication study by Gina Owens (now Gina Gomez de la Cuesta) and her colleagues at Cambridge University. The manual was initially written for research purposes, and not to describe the usual procedures such as setting up and running LEGO Clubs at my office. In fact, the authors and I debated whether to publish it at all since we did not want other therapists and educators to think that there was only one way to do LBT. Following publication of the two first outcome studies (LeGoff & Sherman, 2006; LeGoff, 2004), and then after Gina's doctoral dissertation was published (Owens, *et al*, 2008), we were receiving quite a few requests for additional details about the methods, including requests for workshops and for a training manual. One of Gina's supervisors, Sir Simon Baron Cohen, who was by far the most visible member of our LBT group, strongly supported the publication of the manual that was used by Gina for her doctoral research, ostensibly so he could direct all the inquiries to that source. So, it was somewhat reluctantly that we approached a publisher about making the manual available publicly.

Since that time, both Gina (Dr. Gomez de la Cuesta) and I have had requests to do training workshops, speak to the media, and to offer guidance to colleagues about setting up and running LEGO Club groups. One of the disconcerting discoveries we have made in doing so is that there are literally hundreds, if not thousands, of LBT groups underway, many of which use the LBT manual as if it were some kind of religious doctrine. This book was written to convey the spirit and day-to-day workings of running LEGO Clubs, which should be child-led, creative, and spontaneous, and not adult-led and based on a manual. Although LEGO Clubs are a form of group therapy (they can be billed to health insurance or funded by school districts as an evidence-based group therapy), for the children and adolescents involved, it is a personally meaningful social group and is based on an existing cultural phenomenon. LEGO construction materials, as was clearly shown in Kief Davidson and Daniel Junge's 2014 documentary film, "Beyond the brick: A LEGO brickumentary," are not toys for many children and adults: LEGO is an artistic medium and cultural phenomenon. Obviously, it is not reasonable or even appropriate for educators or therapists to assume control over LEGO materials as if they were developed for doing LBT. The LEGO Corporation has invested many decades of research and creativity in their product, which is now the top selling play material for children worldwide. In my view, an important component of the success of LEGO as play material, which also lends itself to the purposes of improving social development, is its inherent reliance on synergy as an organizational dynamic.

As was discussed earlier, the most important developmental experience which many children do not fully benefit from is interpersonal synergy. Children who experience life in an autistic way tend to approach life and experience it as individuals without as much of a sense of social identity as is typical. Most children see themselves and understand their experiences as both individuals and as members of social groups: family members, siblings, friends, classmates, neighbors, co-workers, partners, and colleagues. Interpersonal relationships are also accompanied by cultural contexts in the home, school, media, community, workplace, and societal institutions. Most children naturally and intuitively identify with and seek approval from others, build relationships, and communicate with others to creatively participate in sociocultural systems. Most children experience the benefits of participating in sociocultural systems through their family experiences, as well as through classrooms, sports teams, clubs, interactions with neighbors, and in other community settings where they encounter both peers and adults. Children who do not naturally view themselves as part of these sociocultural systems do not benefit from or contribute to them as much as they might, and that is a loss of opportunity for creative self-expression for them and for us.

That is ultimately the goal of LBT: to improve the capacity for neurodiverse individuals to creatively participate in sociocultural systems. There are clear potential benefits for both them and society since diversity and inclusive participation are key elements of the adaptive synergy of all sustainable organic systems, from cells to societies. As an organic and synergistic process, LEGO Clubs cannot and should not be formally manualized; they need to remain adaptable to be sustained and adaptable. In that sense, their LBT needs both structure and creative flexibility. The history of LBT has so far shown that it is able to be adaptable and to grow and change over time, but there are now many instances in which it seems to have become stagnated and lifeless because of overly rigid, formalized approaches to running LEGO Clubs and LBT. Although, like any cultural phenomenon there needs to be some stability and structure based on the history of the methodology, it is also important to accept that tradition but be willing to innovate, and in doing so, allow the participants to experience the power of interpersonal synergy.

Short-Term Goals of LBT and How to Evaluate Outcomes. Given that the overall goal of LBT is to offer experiences of interpersonal synergy to children who might otherwise not have such experiences, there is nonetheless a need to convince parents, schools, and other funding sources of the more immediate, short-term value or benefit of group participation. Despite over twenty years of running LEGO groups and doing outcome research to ascertain its benefits, there has not been a standardized tool for outcome evaluation. This is likely due to two factors: first, there is not a single university-based research group identified with this methodology. Regarding my work, I am not a university professor and do not have any formal university affiliations. Although my colleague, Dr. Gina Gomez de la Cuesta, conducted her initial research as part of her doctoral thesis at Cambridge University, she is now a full-time clinician, not a researcher. There has been some attention paid to LBT by university-based research groups, most notably Barry Wright at York-Sheffield University in the UK (Wright, *et al,* 2017), but he has recently retired. The other reason there has not been a single, standardized outcome measure for LBT is the nature of the goal.

Benefitting from the experience of interpersonal synergy in sociocultural systems is nothing like what most outcome studies attempt to measure. As was discussed at length in the recent critique of ABA approaches (LeGoff, 2023), creating objective measures of intervention outcomes is based on how we think about children and their development. Education and therapy are simply extensions of the overall societal process of preparing our offspring for taking on the challenges of sustaining and growing our sociocultural systems. It is important to remind ourselves that interpersonal relationships and culture are the sources of human survival, and now include the survival of the entire system of life on our planet. The origin and continued basis for all human society is interpersonal synergy. Without it, there would be no families, no communities, no technology, no science, no industry, and no civilization. Of course, it is likely that life on the planet would continue without us, but that is less likely an outcome than that human technology and economic systems will persist without the benefit of interpersonal relationships.

The dehumanization of society sounds like a very frightening and remote issue, especially in the context of a book about children playing with LEGO. To make it seem more immediately relevant, however, one need only consider the implications of using radical behaviorism as the basis for child development and education. B.F. Skinner wrote a fictional account of a utopian society (Skinner, 1948) in which civilizations were no longer based on democratic principles and the ideals of individual freedom to participate in societal decision-making. Skinner based these ideas and this vision on his assertion that no organisms, including humans, acted because of internal decision-making, but that their volitional actions (operants) were the result of past experiences of rewards and punishments, operant conditioning (Skinner, 1938). He argued that free will and the capacity for individual decision-making in choosing our actions was just as much an illusion for humans as it was for the pigeons and rats he studied in his laboratory. While Skinner's vision of a utopia in which societal decisions were determined by behavior analytic technology—using reinforcement schedules like those used to shape the behavior of laboratory animals—was never popularized, although it has been used as the basis for several experimental communities which were initiated in the US between 1953 and 1973 (Kuhlmann, 2005; Kincade, 1973). For many who have experienced intensive behavioral intervention programs which are typically implemented simultaneously in the home, classroom, and community, the reality of having all a child's actions determined by the orchestrated rewards (and lack of rewards), including the providing or withholding of "social attention" (i.e., interaction with parents, siblings, friends, classmates, etc.), was a reality, not a hypothetical thought experiment.

Skinner himself was not a clinician or educator and did not study human subjects in his research. He was also not formally trained as a scientist and did not have the benefit of understanding the basics of the scientific method, or the goals of science. Despite the field of ABA being entirely based on the theory and methods of Skinner, there has been a powerful and persisting influence of behavior analysts on the diagnosis of autism, its methods of intervention, and the research methods used to determine the benefits of interventions (LeGoff, 2023). The problem with that situation is clear: ABA itself is not, in fact, a form of scientific inquiry, nor is it a field of science, education, or child psychology. The use of unobtrusive behavioral observation and rewards (positive reinforcement) are used by behavior analysts, but were in fact developed by behavioral psychologists, who are a discipline within the field of psychology, which is a form of scientific inquiry.

Child and educational psychologists use various sorts of measures to assess the developmental and educational progress of children, as well as to evaluate the benefits of individual services plans and education plans, and to assess the costs and benefits of educational and therapeutic programs. While it is important to assess the value of programs or specific intervention methods using group-based outcomes, it is also important to evaluate the costs and benefits of an individual program for a given child and family. While the approaches to program or treatment outcome evaluation and individual progress may overlap in some instances, it is important to keep in mind the important differences: one approach is designed to assess the value of a methodology, and the other is designed to improve the life experience and potential capacity of a child.

With respect to the life experience of children, which is an outcome which is difficult to measure, but importantly, measuring it may not be entirely necessary if a program is voluntary and is designed from the outset to be a positive experience. Noncompliance and "escape-maintained behavior," are common topics in ABA-based interventions for a reason: they are adult-directed and designed with the intention of ignoring the child's experience. Radical behaviorism and ABA are explicitly based on Skinner's assertion that human and other animal experiences of life are not relevant to their decisions and actions. Due to this assertion, behavior analysts are uniformly committed to the view that a child's behavior should be determined by their reinforcement histories, and not their own decisions, choices, preferences, ideas, attachments, attitudes, or beliefs. These are all what Skinner, and his followers refer to as "mentalistic," terms, and which are distractions from the real sources of human behavior, environmental contingencies.

The view espoused here is that the only reason life exists at all is that organisms have some internal ability to choose their actions. Organisms exist as distinct from inert matter because they have the capacity to use their internal structure and internal synergistic dynamics to act in adaptable ways. If organisms could not choose for themselves what to do next, they would not exist. That is the basic premise of allowing children, autistic or otherwise, to choose how to participate in sociocultural systems. Of course, as in all ecosystems, in human sociocultural systems, the range of options from which children choose their actions is largely determined by their genetics and their environments. While Skinner and behavior analysts view the actions of organisms as more or less random prior to being influenced by rewarding or punishing experiences, the fields of ethology, theoretical biology, systems theory, and anthropology have shown that the actions of organisms, including humans, is never random.

The important and under-estimated work of the Russian physiologist and physician, Nikolai Bernstein (1947/2020; 1926/2020; 1948/1996; 1967), is relevant in this respect in that his work showed how individual actions are created by the internal dynamic operations of organisms: actions are the synergistic outcomes of the complex inner operations of organisms. This view is also clear in the works of Bernstein's friend and colleague, Lev Vygotsky (1967; 1933/1978), and other members of the Vygotsky Circle (Shvarts & Bakker, 2019), such as Alexander Luria (Luria, 2002; 1973). Bernstein's work on the theory and neurophysiology of movement demonstrated that actions themselves are necessarily synergistic outcomes of complex internal processes which cannot be determined by environmental conditions. His findings disputed the classical conditioning model being put forward by the more influential Soviet-era researcher, Ivan Pavlov (1941; 1927), and the subsequent works of Skinner. His findings supported the observations and theories of constructivists like Vygotsky and Jean Piaget (1962a), who was unfortunately not able to access either Vygotsky or Bernstein's writings until much later due to the Soviet blockade of scientific and cultural communication with non-Soviet nations (known at the time as the Iron Curtain). In the constructivist view, learning and development are synonymous with both the child's choosing how to participate in their physical and sociocultural environments and the facilitation of insights and skills provided by parents, teachers, mentors, and peers in those environments. This process was described by Vygotsky as creating the Zone of Proximal Development, and by the American follower of both Vygotsky and Piaget, Jerome Bruner, as scaffolding (1986; 1973).

The zone of proximal development and scaffolding are both constructivist conceptualizations of learning and development which reflect synergistic dynamics. As the main proponent of the works of Nikolai Bernstein today, Mark Latash (2021; 2016; 2010; 2008) has described the relationship between the cognitive processes necessary for generating volitional movement and for the acquisition of skilled actions in ways which give important insights into the nature of learning and understanding in general. Insight or understanding of concepts and being able to use knowledge and understanding has been conceptualized from a statistical (Bayesian inference) and artificial intelligence or robotics way by Karl Friston (Friston, *et al*, 2017; Friston, 2010; Friston & Stephan, 2007) as the *free energy principle.*

This model, however, fits artificial intelligence and machine learning much better than organic systems, since the goal of machine learning is to reduce unknowns by determining or fixing degrees of freedom (degrees of freedom is the statistical term for variables in a system with unassigned or unknown values), while the goal of organic systems is adaptability, which necessarily involves both stability and flexibility, such that degrees of freedom remain undetermined and even increased by the system. Increasing degrees of freedom will be the subject of another book, but for now, the basic premise is that organisms have the potential to be synergistically creative in ways that result in emergences—conditions and organizations of energy and matter which did not previously exist. A simple example is the process of reproduction, which is not the same as inert matter replication because new organisms are not identical with their parent organisms, and this is a characteristic built into organic systems at the genetic level and through life experience and learning.

What this foray into theories of science and epistemology boils down to is that organisms, including humans, can choose how they participate in their ecosystems. It is a healthy and normal reaction of organisms, in fact, to rebel against external forces which restrict their ability to determine their own degrees of freedom, or freedom to choose how to think and act. This was the central—and often overlooked—insight and finding of the work of Jack Brehm and his colleagues (Miron & Brehm, 2006; Brehm, 1993; Brehm & Brehm, 1986; Brehm, 1966; Brehm & Cohen, 1962). Psychological reactance theory describes this basic principle in human interpersonal and sociocultural terms, but the theory can be applied to a much wider range of biological systems and ecosystems. What Brehm was describing as a familiar and recognizable phenomenon in adolescents and young adults—rebellion against conformity and against the assertion of control by external influences over individual decision-making and choices—is a fundamental characteristic of organisms and organic systems: they are designed to creatively participate in ecosystems, not to be determined by them.

If we go back to the short-term goals of LBT, we can gain some insight from the first measures used to evaluate its efficacy in terms of improving social competence (LeGoff, 2004). In that study, there were three outcome measures identified which were designed to reflect an overall construct of social competence: self-initiated social contact with peers, the duration of social interactions, and the frequency of potentially interfering or stigmatizing actions. In the case of the first measure, which was defined simply as the number of times in a fixed period during which a child approached other children without adult prompting and initiated social interaction and/or communication, it clearly reflects this idea of freedom of self-determination which is literally the opposite of the behaviorist goal of compliance with adult prompting and adult-controlled reinforcement schedules. Frequency of observed self-initiated contact with peers, however, has limitations as a measurable goal since it is required to be exhibited within the period of observation. If a child improves in their willingness to engage with peers and is successful in interactions with peers, the frequency of those contacts as an objective measure, is as likely to decrease as it is to increase. As was found in that original study, there was at least a clear asymptote after the first 12 weeks of the study: the participants improved initially, and then their rates of self-initiated contact with peers leveled off.

This limitation appears to be more of a problem for group-based research outcomes, however, rather than for individual intervention outcomes since those observations can occur over a much longer time frame. The number of self-initiated contacts with peers during free play can be recorded over a period of a week or more, both at baseline and at outcome, which reduces the problem created by the fact that successfully initiated social interactions are self-limiting in terms of their frequency. Anyone who has been at a successful dinner party or at a large professional conference can attest that our best efforts to initiate contact with peers usually results in a compromise between how many people we can interact with, and how satisfying and meaningful those interactions end up being. There does seem to be some value, none-theless, in keeping track of frequency of child-initiated contacts since most socially competent individuals do seem to find the right balance of num-ber of contacts and meaningfulness of interactions: too few is not ideal, and neither is too many. Using some form of local norm based on typical peer observations—e.g., classmates, or neighboring children in a community—should give parents, therapists, and educators a good sense of what the typical range of rates of self-initiated contact is for a given setting (e.g., classroom, lunchroom, playground, or neighborhood).

The second measure of social competence included in LeGoff (2004) was the mean duration of social interactions with peers during free periods. This measure is also self-limiting because of the maximum duration of free periods, but within that framework, it is less susceptible to the automatic regulation of the operation than frequency of contacts. This was what was observed in that study as well: duration of interactions continued to increase at both 12 weeks and 24 weeks of LBT participation. The use of a measure of central tendency, the mean, as opposed to a measure of maximal achievement helps somewhat in both describing the outcome and avoiding the risk of illusory regressions. That is a problem with many forms of goal setting as they relate to subjective experiences like social interactions with peers, or even academic skills such as amount of time spent reading, doing homework, or practicing a skill: quan-tity does not equal quality. If we use a couple of obvious examples, such as getting into fights with other children on the playground or being rigid and repetitive in practicing a musical instrument, it is easy to see that spending a lot of time doing something does not necessarily mean a child is improving in some meaningful way.

In the case of social development, though, the quality of interactions is necessarily tied to how well a child is engaging with other children, who themselves can choose to continue or stop a playful interaction. If a child sustains an interaction with peers who are not otherwise constrained to engage with that child by adult influences, then something positive must be going on—regardless of how we might subjectively perceive that interaction. In other words, interacting with peers is adaptable regardless of whether we adults think it is appropriate or not. That has been an important lesson for myself and my colleagues, as well as for many of the parents of LEGO Club participants. Appropriateness of interactions are top-down behavioral defini-tions. Fun for LEGO Club participants is defined by the participants, not the adults. Aside from the self-limiting time parameters of periods of free play, the mean duration of social interactions with peers does appear to be the single best measure of social competence that is both easy to record (a stopwatch, a piece of paper or other data recording system, and a person to record them is all that is needed) and meaningful in terms of short-term observable goals (satisfying the requirements of both insurance carriers and school districts).

Finally, the third short-term outcome measure of social competence used in LeGoff (2004) was based on parent ratings of the rates and prevalence of stereotyped movements and idiosyncratic interests. This seems to be the weakest of the three measures and was influenced by the emphasis at the time on using therapeutic interventions to address the observable behaviors of autistic conditions. Defining these actions was not even possible, since there is naturally a wide range of possible idiosyncratic actions. What was used as a measure was one scale of the Gilliam Autism Rating Scale (*GARS*, Gilliam, 1995), which is a measure that can be completed by parents or teachers. There are also now many other standardized and norm-referenced measures of social development and of observed "autistic behaviors." For obvious reasons, it is not recommended that parents, educators, or therapists consider adopting the authoritarian and shortsighted view of behaviorists that being autistic is a behavior problem, and that helping autistic children to meet their developmental goals involves decreasing or increasing the duration and/or frequency of target behaviors.

What is recommended is that adults in any child's life pay attention to the potential impact of the ways that a child attempts to participate—or avoids participating—in sociocultural contexts, and the results of those attempts. Observing children during free play provides a wealth of information about their established and emerging social norms, hierarchies, and culturally specific modes of communication, both verbal and nonverbal. Play is an inherently creative process, but it also reflects the culture in which it occurs, so there are necessarily both consistent features of play as well as variables and flexibility. Inclusion of diversity in play groups is also normal and typical, in fact, children show a greater interest in and willingness to engage with diverse peers than adults do. It is often through adult influences that children begin to adopt the rigidities and biases of their culture, which are often broken down and assimilated during play. For instance, adults are less inclined to engage socially with members of different ethnic or cultural backgrounds unless they have a clear point of identification and common interest, such as having children in the same classroom, being fans of the same professional sports teams, or working on a mutual project together.

Parents of children who exhibit difficulties with social adjustment often naturally hold others responsible, including the children, parents, or teaching staff involved. That may in fact be a reasonable position, but it is not an adaptive one. If a child appears different from their peers in some way, that may be perceived as due to an ethnic or cultural difference, or it may be perceived as an individual's choices and conduct (Wainryb, *et al*, 2004; Wainryb, Shaw & Maianu, 1998). Importantly, while children's views regarding their peers' behavior changes over time, consistent with changes in their moral reasoning abilities, most children distinguish between being different and being inappropriate or argumentative. While most children seem to be tolerant and accepting of cultural and ethnic differences—especially if that is what is modeled by their parents and other adults—but are less so of what the perceive to be self-interested deviations, or self-motivated disruptive behavior (Verkuyten & Killen, 2021).

While some parents and teachers may feel it is unnecessary and potentially stigmatizing to identify neurodiverse children in the classroom, this research suggests that it may be helpful if managed in an appropriate way. The tolerance that other children show towards neurodiverse peers may depend on how their actions are perceived as either an inherent difference in perspective, or as belief discrepancy and dissenting practices which are chosen by the neurodiverse child. Just as importantly, the recognition of diversity and the goal of inclusion is a reciprocal process: both typical and atypical peers should understand that they may have differences in behavior, appearance, and values which are acceptable and normal in that context, even if they are not always consistent with the guidelines and policies being followed by the adults in the room. That is one of the reasons that LEGO Club groups use two different sets of rules: common behavioral expectations, and then the Rules of Cool, which apply to common aspirational goals which are universal to interpersonal actions and communication.

For these and other reasons, acting the same as other children is not a goal of LBT. Acting in ways which foster identification with each other as members of the same group, sharing of ideas and respectful disagreement, joint accomplishment, mutual respect, and exchanging of efforts, time, and resources are goals. Given that all children are born into sociocultural systems in their homes, communities, and schools, it is not necessary to specify as a goal that they should engage in target behaviors, since no specific behavior will be adaptable and valued in all settings and cultures, or even in individual settings at different times. Since sociocultural systems vary and evolve as much as individuals do, what makes more sense is to assess the extent to which a child can sustain their participation in those activities. Frequency of self-initiated contact over a longer period, and mean duration of interaction with peers are therefore still the most reasonable and efficient measures of the overall goal of improving a child's capacity to creatively participate in interpersonal synergy and sociocultural systems.

Long-Term Goals of LBT. While it may seem obvious from the requirements that are inherent in LEGO Club participation—it has a peer-ranked level system (see below)—the long-term goal of LBT should not be defined as being successful in LEGO Club, or for that matter, being successful on the playground. That was an insight which I received by personal communication from an esteemed colleague, Ami Klin. Aside from the obvious benefit of having a positive life experience in the group, participants and their parents should also be able to expect some improvement in longer term quality of life and social competence. Over the years, I have been able to stay in touch with many former group members who have communicated about their current accomplishments vocationally and socially, which is obviously not an objective source of outcome data, though it is certainly encouraging.

In response to Klin's critique of using direct observation of social interaction with peers, the second published outcome study on LBT (LeGoff & Sherman, 2006), used a combination of the Vineland Adaptive Behavior Scales (VABS, Sparrow, *et al*, 1984) and the GARS Social Interaction (SI) scale (Gilliam, 1995). The Vineland, which has been published in its second and third editions by now (Sparrow, *et al*, 2005; Sparrow, *et al*, 2016), is a standardized, operationally defined rating scale (self, parent, and teacher versions are available) of adaptive social, communication, and self-care skills. In the study itself, the emphasis was on the VABS Socialization Domain (VABS-SD), which was shown to have improved by two standard deviations (mean change = +20.68) over a period of three years for 60 children who participated in LBT, which was significantly more than a comparable group of 57 children who received equivalent forms of other therapies (mean change = +10.77). On the GARS-SI, there was also a significant improvement, as indicated by a decrease in SI scores, over the same three-year period.

Overall, the VABS appears to be a better long-term outcome measure since it is not specific to "autistic behavior," or being classified as autistic, which is the case for the GARS, and because it can be used to assess social competency across the lifespan (the VABS-3 has been validated and has online electronic versions with updated norms for all age groups including older adults). One of the built-in characteristics of the LEGO Club model in its more recent iterations is the role that participants can play who have graduated from the group by reaching the highest level (see below). These participants are what is referred to in the LEGO Club as LEGO Legends, and they attend groups as peer mentors. These are children, adolescents and young adults who volunteer to participate in groups because they still enjoy participating and because they see the value in helping other children achieve their level of social competence. Aside from that direct indication of social development, as is discussed below, most children who succeed in LEGO Club naturally tend to show competence in participating in other sociocultural systems at school, at home, and in their communities.

These are developmental and personal achievements which are difficult to quantify on an individual basis, but which are also obvious and meaningful to the children and their families. For the purposes of research, it may be helpful to quantify these accomplishments, however, up to this point, neither my colleagues nor I have felt the need to do so. In addition to participating in other social systems, additional outcome measures such as achieving independent living status, economic self-sufficiency, personal relationships, and parental status would also be important data which has yet to be collected or compared with non-participant controls. Readers who are themselves involved in clinical research are invited to consider looking at these types of long-term outcomes. For the purposes of this book, however, individual outcomes which include independent adaptive functioning are encouraged, and are easily assessed in young adult clients.

There are numerous alternatives to the VABS-3 currently available, such as the Adaptive Behavior Assessment Scales, Third Edition (ABAS-3; Harrison & Oakland, 2015). Aside from having age-norms from early childhood to late adulthood, the ABAS-3 and VABS-3 are also both correlated with autistic symptom ratings and cognitive abilities. This is logical since cognitive abilities and psychopathology or severity of autistic features impact adaptive functioning, and in the end, in addition to improved quality of life, adaptive functioning is the goal of implementing interventions and supports. Since quantifying cognitive abilities using IQ tests or symptomatology using behavioral measures are both ethically and clinically questionable ways of assessing an individual's life experience and functioning, the benefits of LBT can be restricted to just standardized measures of adaptation.

CHAPTER 4

SETTING UP A LEGO CLUB

LEGO as a System. As mentioned above, LEGO itself is a system of interlocking pieces or bricks which have both unique and general purposes in terms of both representational or symbolic functions and then pragmatic, structural functions. While it is not important for the group participants to have a group leader who is an expert on LEGO materials, since the group leader is also often the person ultimately responsible for acquiring the materials, budgeting for the LEGO Club acquisitions, and maintaining the materials, they should be generally familiar with the history of LEGO, its system, its themes and genres, and the ways that LEGO can be used in various forms of construction play and creative expression. LEGO is quintessentially synergistic in the sense that it has a stable system and traditions (including the LEGO Corporation itself, which has been owned and operated by four generations of a single Danish family), which are also widely diverse, innovative, and creative. For most children, their introduction to LEGO building materials involves following basic block connecting and set-building techniques, often taught to them by parents, peers, or older siblings.

This stable base of operations is then gradually added to as children acquire the skills which enable them to become innovative (e.g., modifying sets), and then creative (designing and building their own sets). Innovating with LEGO involves modifying a set or construction or using pieces in unique ways to improve, specialize, or personalize them visually or functionally. Creating involves coming up with unique constructions or ways to use LEGO visually and functionally. While it is not necessary that group leaders know all there is to know about this complex system and its history, they should understand the basics of how the system operates, and how children are able to participate with it, both individually and in groups. Reading this manual, the previous manual, as well as some of the other literature about LBT, is a good start, but inevitably, those interested in starting and running LEGO Clubs (LBT groups) should watch some of the more general media (e.g., the LEGO Brickumentary; Youtube.com/lego+stop+motion) and become familiar with the LEGO websites and fan sites (e.g., LEGO.com and Bricklink.com).

Selecting Group Members. Aside from creating a holding environment or boundary which establishes the capacity for the LEGO Club as a dynamic system to determine its own internal degrees of freedom (the variables of what happens in a play group), one of the most important characteristics of a successful group is mutual identification and shared values. The process of group member selection can vary a lot depending on the organizational context and professionals involved. In my experience of running groups, the members were either referred to my private practice for outpatient evaluation and treatment (individual, family, and group therapy), or they were seen at their school (private or public) in which a LEGO Club group had been established to meet the needs of the students. In a private clinic setting, it is up to the therapist, the child, and their parents to decide whether to give LEGO Club a try, and if there is more than one group ongoing, which group to attend. Some private clinics offer a set number of sessions for a given group of participants, e.g., 12 sessions, and all the participants start and end the LBT at the same time. In other settings, there may be more than one group and they are ongoing, but parents or the children's schools will fund a certain number of group sessions, and continuing or ending therapy is based on some pre-determined criteria based on goal attainment.

Group members tend to progress more quickly in achieving relevant social competence goals when they can identify with and collaborate with peers in the group whom they perceive as being like them, which was the basis for the decision to host the first joint LEGO-based therapy sessions. The experience of interacting with another peer whom a participant experiences as being "like me," is not entirely determined by external characteristics like age, gender, or cognitive and language development. Many different interpersonal characteristics are required for children and adults to perceive others as potential collaborators, and friends. Many socially competent individuals experience a sense of interpersonal bonding or relationship with others who disclose personal information and express emotions. In my experience, while disclosure and shared emotions can be important in enriching interpersonal connections, most autistic children (especially boys), experience interpersonal attachment to others who share their interests and with whom they can collaborate on personally relevant activities or tasks. In other words, they bond over doing things together, not by sharing personal information or talking about their emotional or interpersonal experiences.

LEGO Club enhances social competence by providing experiences of interpersonal synergy, which means learning the value of working together. While not all a group's activities are going to be synergistic, just like any other system, it will operate in ways that maintain the stability or homeostasis of the group, rather than its growth or replication. When I look back on how LEGO Club first started, however, it is not surprising how quickly the first couple of participants became dozens of participants, and the first dyad became many separate groups: that is a natural, organic outcome of a synergistic system. I have also observed many other LEGO Club groups which were either static and did not grow and adapt, or they resulted in immediate conflicts and were not sustainable. These failed groups or persistently maladaptive ones are not the result of an absence of interpersonal synergy but reflect the presence of antergistic influences; factors which work against the values and benefit of the members.

The most obvious mistakes I have seen that result in antergistic dynamics are when adults who do not understand the basic principles of interpersonal synergy and the goal of LEGO Club in increasing the participant's experience of interpersonal synergy are put in charge. In these groups, the goals of the group are defined by the therapist/leader, and not from the perspectives of the group members, and they emphasize externally defined behavioral objectives. The values of mutual benefit, creative sharing, and collaborative achievement are de-emphasized in favor of the institutional goals of compliance and rule-following with the goal of increasing the rates of behaviors that are defined by unfamiliar social and communication norms. Using operant strategies to encourage a child to behave *as if* they were more neurotypical or *as if* they had more common interests and values, inevitably devalues that child's natural interests and values.

What motivates most children to play, and thereby acquire the knowledge and skills of their culture, is an innate affinity with those around them, not some external reward. It is not helpful to try to replace a child's low social motivation using other rewards, especially if the activities involved are experienced as foreign and are not recognized as being potentially part of their emerging sense of self. Positive reinforcement or adult-enforced rules are reminders to neurodiverse children of their differences and their struggles with experiencing included and part of a synergistic system. They do not lead to identification with others; they enforce separateness and the experience of being a foreigner in your own home. They can also elicit psychological reactance ("oppositional behavior"), social avoidance, and learned helplessness, which are the results of antergistic and maladaptive interpersonal dynamics.

Skills and creativity. Nikolai Bernstein's studies on movement and skill acquisition provide important insights about the process by which our brains internalize and then determine the degrees of freedom of action. As mentioned above, this model has also been shown to apply to how we can internalize the degrees of freedom of concepts (Latash, 2021). If we consider a movement or a construct as having both a stable structure—the body or the cognitive facility—as well as variables which describe options for the action of that structure, that is what Bernstein was attempting to describe. Bernstein understood that what distinguished living organisms from inorganic matter was the existence of options or choices about how that organism could operate which were internal to the organism. What Bernstein described as redundant degrees of freedom were not just the lucky happenstance of being a complex organism and having multiple ways of acting upon the environment, they were necessary for evolution and the adaptability of all life forms. Without redundant degrees of freedom, and the internal capacity to choose how to achieve future goals—what to do next—organisms would lack diversity and flexibility of action, which would be just as fatal as a lack of genetic diversity and flexibility. It is a basic principle of being able to survive on our stably unstable planet.

While Skinner conceived of skill acquisition as the elimination of variability within a given environmental context—allowing the environment to determine the optimal action in each circumstance—both Bernstein and Vygotsky described skill acquisition as the internalization of a set of variables which could be used creatively to achieve an internal goal. In other words, rather than outcomes shaping our behavior so that it appears skillful, through a combination of self-initiated trial and error and modeling of observed actions, children shape the events around them to become consistent with their intended outcomes. By identifying with others, most children benefit from the advantage of both sharing a set of values which allow them to become aligned with mutual goals (they enjoy and want what we want), and they are willing to play at doing what others around them do. This is the basis for what is commonly observed in children playing: they are teaching themselves how to participate in the sociocultural synergy around them. Those are the skills that their society values.

Just as importantly, though—and something that is not so evident in the work of Bernstein, or Latash—children learn how to be creative. That is somewhat inevitable in the process of skill acquisition, but the extent to which flexibility, innovation, and creativity are evident in a child's play and development, will vary according to the activity, the level of the child's skill development, and variables of the setting in which the play occurs. Sports and music are good examples of culturally specific skills which combine skill acquisition with creative self-expression, but these dynamics can also be applied to any cultural skill such as language proficiency, math and logical reasoning, and interpersonal competence. When a child kicks a ball or plucks a string on an instrument, they are not just acquiring a behavior or demonstrating a movement: they are acquiring the insight that they control the variables or degrees of freedom of that action. Simultaneously with getting something right—like putting two LEGO bricks together—a child is learning about the many ways they can choose from to achieve that outcome. This is much more than simply learning from our mistakes, which is an idea that presumes that there is ultimately a single ideal way of achieving a goal. What Bernstein showed us was that there may be an almost infinite number of ways of getting something right. The true notion of a skill involves the internal capacity to both choose an outcome (based on our values), as well as to choose how we arrive at that outcome. A beginner in any form of self-expression may be focused on modeling their actions and outcomes on skills demonstrated by others, but as they improve, they will increasingly individualize and vary their approach, the way a more skilled artist or musician adds innovation and nuance to their work.

For autistic children, the skill acquisition process in development does not benefit as much from the shortcuts offered by modeling and imitation—the scaffolding provided by parents, siblings, peer mentors, teachers, and coaches—and therefore, they do not have the same depth to their *zone of proximal development*. The ZPD concept was used by Vygotsky to describe the difference between what a typical child may be able to acquire in terms of skill or knowledge on their own, versus that which could be achieved by using models. Due to their decreased level of social identification and shared value, autistic children are less inclined to respond to modeling by internalizing observed skillful actions, and thereby to benefit from scaffolding. This includes the modeling of creative processes since scaffolding not only allows a child to observe a skill, but how to innovate and be creative in executing that skill. These processes are emphasized in the LEGO Club in ways which are naturally beneficial.

LEGO materials and the level system of LBT both provide support for feeling at home and not having to live up to foreign expectations or social norms, as well as introducing the participants to positive experiences of scaffolding, joint accomplishment, and shared creativity. The participants themselves often express insight about the potential benefit they experience in the presence of other children's LEGO creations or exhibitions of LEGO-based skills: "I could do that!" That insight is not simply about recognizing their LEGO-building capacity but expresses a shared value ("I could do that because I would enjoy doing it and it would be worthwhile and valued by others"), and a sense of shared identity ("I could do that because I am like them"). Just as LEGO materials reflect both form and function, the shared activities in LEGO Club involve first a focus on the skills of putting sets together—dictated by form—and then innovative and creative actions with those forms. The children do not just acquire the skilled actions of LEGO builders, they acquire the concepts of how bricks work together—how bricks act in synergistic ways—and then how they can collaborate with their peers in synergistic, creative ways.

Although many children will not express their insights about how participating in synergistic LEGO-building, or in a synergistic interpersonal activity, has benefitted them (although some certainly have done), what is evident is their increased motivation for social interaction in a range of play and learning activities. It may be somewhat of a struggle for some children initially to give up their goals of building LEGO by themselves, but if they are prepared in advance for the trade-off of individual achievement for the benefits of shared achievement, they often adapt to it in surprising ways. It is a common experience for parents, educators, and therapists to observe a child begrudgingly agree to give LEGO Club a try, and then quickly become engrossed by it, and insist on getting to LEGO Club on time, or early, and never want to miss a session. They will ask to have playdates with their new LEGO Club friends and ask if they can come to groups more often and bring their classmates or siblings with them. This is not the result of a single factor, like self-efficacy, skill acquisition, or social identity; it is a synergistic outcome of an organic system made up of diverse elements.

Synergy and antergy are opposing outcomes or epiphenomena resulting from the dynamic operations within systems. They can be thought of as a gradient, from adaptive and creative to maladaptive and destructive, and most systems over time may experience periods of synergistic growth, antergistic deterioration, or more stable homeostasis. For children, the natural expectation is that they will participate in their sociocultural environment in ways which lead to growth and development, but at times, all children experience periods of regression or decline in response to stressors. As they do, they typically need to become resilient and adaptable, and thereby developing strengths to help them overcome future life stressors. Under most conditions, as the constructivist theorists and researchers have described, children benefit from combining their internal and external resources in synergistic ways, the outcome of which is often innovative and adaptable skill development. In other situations, however, a child's inner resources for adaptive coping are thwarted, frustrated, or ignored by their social environment, which leads to negative outcomes like mistrust of others, poor self-efficacy, learned helplessness, and reactance.

For children with autistic traits, these outcomes are more likely due to the initial absence of typical sociality—identification with others and innate sense of shared values and interests. Once single factors within a system, such as a child in a family, or student in a classroom, begin to have a negative influence on a child's willingness to participate in that system, they can trigger an escalating sequence of factors, a negative cascade effect. Curiosity about what seems foreign or different if not accepted as such can become suspicion, and then mistrust, and finally hostility. Anxiety or hesitancy about participating can be misinterpreted as aloofness, and then stubbornness, selfishness, and then antisocial attitudes. Being low on trait sociality, or autistic, is not an antisocial trait, any more than being low on musicality or being low on math ability means a person hates music or math. Children who have an innate difference, however, can be pushed in antergistic directions if others are not understanding of their experience and point of view. Alternatively, as we try to do in LEGO Club, we invite children to share their different experiences and to feel valued for them, which leads them in synergistic directions, working together towards self-expression, growth, and having a sense of shared, mutual value. LEGO materials themselves—bricks and ideas for how to combine them—reflect this synergistic dynamic inherently, and they invite children to engage in synergistic building.

LEGO can also be used to express antergy in ways that can overcome it. Children can experience destructive impulses, and symbolically express them through their intuitive awareness of resentment and disaffiliation by demolishing others or their own creations. It can be a therapeutic process for children to destroy and then rebuild sets or creations, being innovative and creative in the process. That process expresses hope that dysfunctional interpersonal dynamics can also be reversed. In LEGO groups, I have often sparked a sense of recognition and shared this experience with the members by purposely destroying LEGO sets or creations. I have just tossed LEGO sets in the air or crushed them with my hands in apparent frustration or ill will towards my own or someone else's work. Then, rather than lingering on that negative emotion, I move straight on to redeeming myself by starting the rebuilding process, but I invariably need the help of my LEGO friends, so we rebuild better synergistically.

Form, function, and symbolic representation. While a brick is sometimes just a brick, as an element of the LEGO system also can have a specific form which gives it functional value but is also useful for symbolic representation. This dual role of bricks is both an obvious characteristic of LEGO pieces, for example, a mini-fig head, with or without a face, is also a single-stud round brick, and a simple four stud square brick can also be a head, with or without a face. Sometimes a piece is a head and sometimes it is just a building block, and it is the child's playful decisions and choices that determine which. In that sense, children learn that they can choose not only what to do with the world around them, but how to think about it: objects and actions as well as ideas are becoming accessible to them as building blocks for their growing internal cognitive system. Symbolic representation is a key part of cognitive development which leads children towards understanding culture and how culture imbues certain objects, actions, and ideas with value. In this way, LEGO materials are like language, which is made up of elements which are at times functional, and at other times symbolic or representational, but they gain meaning and value only within the context of shared experiences: interpersonal relationships and culture.

Latash (2021) explains how understanding an idea is based on the same synergistic operations as generating a movement. In that sense, LEGO bricks are a good analogy for neurons and brain systems: symbolic representations are built from diverse elements and take on both new purposes, and functions, as well as new meanings, depending on how they are combined. While the idea of symbolic representation in the brain is well established in cognitive neuroscience, the role of synergistic operation of brain systems in generating movement originated with Bernstein (1947/2020), and that work only became more widely available due to Latash's translation of it into English. Latash has since pursued Bernstein's ideas about how the brain and body function synergistically to generate movements and acquire skills towards a more general theory on the role of synergy in cognition.

While the concept of interpersonal synergy has been around for many centuries, it is only very recently that cognitive and organizational scientists have begun to explore synergistic systems models of both individual and group cognition and decision-making. Kozlowski and Chau (2012) and Koslowski, *et al*, (2013) have described how emergences—new ideas and new processes—in the workplace are generated by both bottom-up (individuals and their interactions) and top-down (the group dynamic as a whole) synergistic properties. They have also outlined how these systems dynamics and their outcomes can be studied by organizational psychologists. Curseu, *et al* (2015) have extended Koslowski and Chau's model which is based on the work of Patrick Laughlin on synergistic group dynamics and problem-solving (Laughlin, Carey & Kerr, 2008; Laughlin & Barth, 1981; Laughlin & Sweeney, 1977). The goal of this line of research has been to directly examine the impact of group dynamics on individual decision-making competencies, which Goos, Galbraith, and Renshaw (2002) described as a *collaborative zone of proximal development* (CZPD). This is a variation of Vygotsky's initial description of the ZPD, which is characteristic of learning and development at the interpersonal level, which includes the influence of group dynamics. In this view, the emergent construct of an organization—like a business entity, or a team—has simultaneous and reciprocal influences on individuals as well as on smaller groups such as dyads, triads, or work groups.

Vygotsky described the dyadic influence of a child and parent, teacher, sibling, or peer in advancing the cognitive development of the child through modeling of skills and demonstrating effective decision-making using concepts that the child had not yet achieved as creating a zone of proximal development (ZPD, Vygotsky, 1933/1978). Bruner (1986) also described this process as scaffolding, which involved a similar dynamic involving one-on-one tutoring or teaching of a child to confer cognitive insights which could then be used by the child to improve their decision-making and problem-solving. In the original study demonstrating the process of scaffolding, by Wood, Bruner, and Ross (1976), the authors used a construction play activity—a pyramid made from complex interconnecting blocks. An adult tutored the child learning how to use the blocks. The tutor did not solve the design and construction problems for the child participants, but gave support and pointed out when the child had missed something or made a mistake: "… a tutor seeks to teach children 3, 4 and 5 yr to build a particular three-dimensional structure that requires a degree of skill that is initially beyond them … A great deal of early problem solving by the developing child is of this order." Wood *et al*, go on to outline the unique and critical value of these sort of student-teacher relationships not only for the classroom but for child development in general, and thereby, for our species as a whole:

> *What distinguishes man as a species is not only his capacity for learning, but for teaching as well. It is the main aim of this paper to examine some of the major implications of this interactive, instructional relationship between the developing child and his elders for the study of skill acquisition and problem solving* (Wood, Bruner & Ross, 1976).

According to Laughlin, and then as demonstrated by the research of Merrilyn Goos, Steve Koslowski, Petru Curseu, and their colleagues, what was not observed and therefore not accounted for by either Vygotsky or Bruner was the additional influence of the group—the classroom, team, or organization—on the learning and problem-solving of individuals. Laughlin, *et al* (2008; 2006; 2002) established the superiority of small group problem-solving on complex number-letter tasks, which demonstrated an emergent quality of group dynamics over teacher-student interactions in conceptual problem-solving and decision-making. In other words, there is something about learning as a group which is qualitatively better than individual instruction, and that has to do with the synergistic dynamics of the group process. Koslowski and Chao demonstrated that this emergent outcome of adult group dynamics reflects the additional levels within the overall interpersonal system. There is not one level of teacher-student or parent-child relationship, but additional dynamics which reflect both bottom-up (learner-to-learner, sub-group-to-teacher, sub-group-to-larger group influences), and top-down (teacher-to-learner, teacher-to-sub-group, subgroup-to-learner, larger group-to-subgroup, etc.).

Goos, Galbraith, and Renshaw (2002), reported on an extensive, three-year study on math problem-solving and the meta-cognitive processes of high school students. They described how students could improve each other's problem solving through collaborative ZPD, over and above the influence of adult-directed classroom instruction. This peer-group mediated the phenomenon of growth in meta-cognition (problem-solving and decision-making), as described by Laughlin. Koslowski and Chao emphasized the two core conditions for successful emergence in organizational and team relationships as cognition and cohesion (Felin, Koslowski & Chao, 2012). These are essentially the same conditions of collaborative group mental activity with a common goal, also described by Curseu, *et al* (2015), in their findings on adult small group problem-solving efficiency.

Peter Corning, from an evolutionary perspective, has described the importance of collaboration at the individual, group, and species level as a core characteristic of success of the human species, with culture as an important emergent result of cognitive synergy between individuals and at higher orders of social organization. He argues that this is a universal dynamic among species as well as being a necessary characteristic of all adaptable ecosystems, especially sociocultural ones. While Corning's work is viewed as most relevant to theoretical biology, the collaborative dynamics he describes are essentially the same as those described in the organizational psychology literature, and originally, in the writings of the social constructivists, Vygotsky, Piaget, and Bruner, and the theoretical biology of von Bertalanffy's general systems theory. The intra-organismic evidence of the dynamic operations of hierarchically organized systems are probably most objectively described by Nikolai Bernstein's movement studies.

What is most relevant for understanding the therapeutic process involved in LBT is the limitation that low sociality or weak anthropocentrism imposes on some individuals. All children—in fact, all organisms, and even artificially intelligent machines—develop and adapt using internal hierarchical principles involving redundant internal degrees of freedom (choice options in goal-attainment) and synergistic motor-planning and decision-making, internal cognitive and muscle synergies (Latash, 2021; Alessandro, *et al*, 2013). These internal organizational dynamics result in the capacity of systems to be self-sustaining and to grow by learning and acting on flexible problem-solving strategies, but these dynamic operations also apply to external organizations, like families, classrooms, teams, and businesses. As result, these dynamics are also evident in the histories of existing cultures and societies which rely on both individual and group emergences (Muthukrishna, *et al*, 2018; 2016), such as innovation, creativity, and play (Moll & Tomasello, 2007; Tomasello, *et al*, 2005; Tomasello, 1999; 1996). Despite having the capacity to use internal synergistic cognitive and motor synergies, children with weak sociality who do not have an innate sense of shared values and goals with those around them, do not naturally contribute to and benefit from external, sociocultural synergies.

As described above, while not participating in synergistic dynamics on its own is not necessarily detrimental, there are many examples of how the positive dynamics we associate with interpersonal cognitive synergies can become maladaptive. For many children who participate in LBT, especially younger children, they may not have experienced negative social interactions such as feeling misunderstood, excluded, or bullied by peers, or criticized, cajoled, and hounded by parents and professionals at home and in the classroom. Most children who are given a diagnosis of an autistic condition, however, will likely to be exhibiting acquired maladaptive coping strategies which are the hallmarks of interpersonal and sociocultural antergy. It is both improving the developmental, social, and vocational benefits of interpersonal synergy, as well as preventing or reversing the impact of interpersonal antergy, that are the central goals of LBT. Being a member of the LEGO Club is an experience of interpersonal and cultural synergy. Many children might otherwise not benefit from such experiences or have ones that are either not personally relevant or potentially maladaptive and antergistic.

CHAPTER 5

LEGO-BASED THERAPY AS A SOCIOCULTURAL SYSTEM

H</br>istory is an important source of information which can offer more than scientific knowledge and understanding because science is derived from the aggregate of insights of individuals who exist within a given sociocultural context and have their own subjective biases and perspectives. History is a record of events, which can also be presented in subjective ways, but it contains both culture and science, not the other way around. In other words, it is useful to consider the history of science, and less so, the science of history. In human history, what is important to consider with respect to LBT, is the anthropological evolution of interpersonal relationships and culture. Before there was culture, there were families, and before there were families, our ancestors were simply individual organisms. We can go back a long way in our evolutionary history before we encounter pre-human species who did not benefit from culture, and almost back to the origins of life on earth before we find evidence of any pre-human ancestors who were not social. Homo sapiens, in our current form, have been both social and cultural, out of necessity, but also out of design: we are who we have become as species because of our genetic design, and those genes were also selected by sociocultural ecosystem pressures.

Participation in interpersonal relationships and culture—customs and traditions that are passed down from one generation to the next including language, social norms, skills, and technology—are necessary features of adaptive development for children. While social development and many features of culture are assimilated naturally through participation in social systems like the family and community, much of what children acquire in terms of skills needed to become participants in sociocultural systems are acquired through formal educational curriculum in school (or as is more common these days, home-schooling). The research described in the previous chapter on social constructivist models of learning and development, and on interpersonal and cognitive synergy in workgroups and business organizations, presumes typical sociality: the participants in those studies and the individuals for whom their findings are considered relevant are neurotypical and have average levels of sociality. These findings imply that the basis for current models of education and successful participation in most vocations are applicable to anthropocentric humans, not autistic ones.

The use of ABA in homes and classrooms may be considered generally a form of work-around for the problem of being autistic as opposed to neurotypical and anthropocentric, however, the goals and methods of ABA do not directly address the underlying issues. The argument from behavior analysts—and other superficial forms of autism intervention or support—is that they do not need to understand what causes autism since they can use operant conditioning to change autistic behavior. The main flaw with that point of view is that child development and learning as well as adult adaptive functioning require an individual to be an active participant in a sociocultural system; they cannot just behave *as if* they were a part of that system, they need to *be* a part of that system. As was described above and is well described in the works of Tomasello and his colleagues, becoming an active participant in society requires children to identify with and be motivated to participate in sharing knowledge, skills, language, and social norms. These are equally accessible to all children—at least initially—but autistic children do not intuitively understand why these sources of information should be more valuable and important than any others, such as the physical world around them.

Physical, temporal, symbolic and social boundaries. All sustainable systems have boundaries. It is easier to see and understand how a boundary creates an opportunity for the separation of events inside a system from those in its environment. In some cases, boundaries are physical and are put in place from outside the system itself, like fences, hedgerows, border walls, the boards of a hockey rink, the fence around a tennis court, the walls of a building, the skin of a vehicle. There are also boundaries which emerge from the system itself, such as the cell walls, epithelial tissues, exoskeletons, or bark of living organisms. These are obvious in the way they allow what happens inside of them to occur with some independence from what is happening outside. Boundaries allow a system to operate with some degree of freedom from the events in its environment, and in adaptable systems like ecosystems and sociocultural systems, or niches within those systems, the ability for individual organisms to have internal degrees of freedom independent from the environment is a necessity. Through the processes of genetic transmission across generations, as well as through individual experience and learning, the internal conditions of organisms are variable and diverse in relation to the events which challenge them, and that variability and diversity establishes the redundant degrees of freedom necessary for flexible adaptation.

Unlike organic systems like children, physical and sociocultural systems do not have their own internal degrees of freedom: they are fully dependent on the events in the environment of which they are a part. Whether it is an ant hill or an automobile, those are inert physical objects which fully obey the laws of physics. Ecosystems and societies survive and evolve because of the organisms who create them. One of the surprising findings of the history of the evolution of life on our planet and of human culture is the central role of play in that evolution. What we observe around us in both ecosystems and sociocultural systems is the product of skillful manipulation of materials— work—but the original ideas for using materials in adaptable ways, and the skills needed to bring those ideas into reality, originated in play.

Although there are many scientific theories about the functions of play, but if we look towards its history and not just the way that play appears in our sociocultural systems today, we realize that all acquired skills are transmitted across generations through the process of one organism (usually the younger one) playing with the materials and skills of another. What separates the creative learning process associated with play from the necessary adaptive activities of a species participating in its ecosystem is the creation of a boundary which separates the play activity from the events and consequences of its environment. Those boundaries are sometimes obvious like the walls of a playroom, the mesh of a play pen, or fence around a playground, but they can also be temporal, like playtime, recess, or practice, or symbolic, as in the use of toys, costumes, or other materials. What distinguishes play from work is not just the sense of fun or the freedom to be creative, but the physical, temporal, and symbolic boundaries which distinguish it from "real life," or the day-to-day adaptive participation in our physical and sociocultural environment.

The other source of a boundary around play as a system separate from others is social. In human play as with other species, this is a key boundary because it is based on the relationship between individuals, and not on the inner processes of those organisms. Playing together requires that all parties understand and agree that we are, in fact, playing. This is an important feature of LEGO Club because it allows the participants to participate in an "as if" play world without the challenges and consequences of the sociocultural systems "out there," in the classroom or in the community. This is not just a feature of LBT but applies to all forms of intervention designed to help neurodiverse children, and to some extent to all forms of therapy and remedial education in general. Improving a child's capacity to participate in their sociocultural environment should not be focused solely on that child—as it is with many forms of intervention from drug therapies to psychotherapy—or on that child's environment—as is the case with behavioral interventions and parental coaching—but on the relationship between that child and their environment. This means changing not just how a child experiences and thinks about their environment, but that environment's permeability to the child's influence.

The permeability of the boundary between an organism and its environment is another way of describing the extent of reciprocal relatedness between them. As separate systems, they cannot be fully permeable, but as systems with mutual influence they cannot be fully closed from each other, either. Sociality as a genetic and learned trait describes the degree to which an individual is open to the potential benefits of affiliation and collaboration. Keep in mind that a minimal level of sociality is not an indication of pathology in humans—or any other social species—since it is normal and adaptable for us to have a range of expressions of this trait. More innately social individuals, however, will be more motivated and will show a greater degree of reciprocal permeability with their social environment. Highly social children do not need external support or structuring (scaffolding) to benefit from and contribute creatively to their sociocultural systems. Less social children, however, do need to have more structured boundaries and more intensely enjoyable, beneficial experiences of their sociocultural system. Otherwise, they will be content to play on their own, in their own way. That is not necessarily a problem, either, but in our current sociocultural system being left alone to play in your own way is not only just about impossible, but it can also be potentially limiting for the child's advanced educational and vocational opportunities and can limit the extent to which the rest of us can benefit from their unique contributions.

For these reasons, LEGO Club as a therapeutic peer-group experience needs to have boundaries and a structure which helps identify it as an opportunity to play, as well as to replicate many of the features of typical play situations, which are common for all of us, not just children. When any of us play, we tend to do so with others who have a mutual interest and experience a similar sense of benefit. We play in places that are demarcated for the purpose, and we play during time periods which are also demarcated as separate from other daily activities. Giving children a time and a place to play, and peers to play with, is one of the most important challenges we are given as adults. It is also largely the adults who influence what children play with, although to some extent, children naturally choose play materials on their own. For social children, with a high level of identification and shared values with their parents, siblings, and peers, they want to play with what adults show them to be important: the tools and technology of their daily lives.

"Playing with," however, also implies that children are engaged in activities which take the form, if not the goal, or adult activities including the skills, social relationships, roles, language, and communication patterns of typical adult behavior. Becoming like their parents, or other adults, through play, not only serves the purpose of passing down culturally specific skills, social norms, and language, but also demonstrates the value of those children to the adults in their culture ("I'm becoming one of you,"), and contributes to the growth and adaptability of culture. Just as children are unique genetically which benefits the sustainability of their species, their life experiences and playful creativity contribute to the diversity and adaptability of their culture on which their species relies for survival. Adults go to the trouble of creating a time and place for children to play and offering them the materials they need if they do not get them on their own, because children playing is how culture survives, and culture is how humans survive.

What needs to be emphasized for children who are not inherently social is how participating in culturally relevant play can benefit them as well as the rest of us. That is not something that can be designed and constructed as an educational or behavioral intervention because it needs to be part of the organic and growing relationship between a child and others. Just as you cannot construct an organism, you cannot construct social relationships. You cannot make a child participate in their sociocultural environment any more than we can make any animal participate in its natural ecosystem. What we can do, however, is create a safe place and time which are a microcosm of those systems and allow them to play.

Setting and maintaining the semi-permeable boundary of the LEGO Club. Setting the various parameters of LBT in advance is especially important since what happens during the group sessions should be child-led and natural as much as possible. Under the right conditions, the organic change that occurs does need a lot of adult direction, but there are many variables involved in establishing those conditions. Further discussion of some of these variables is provided below, and it is important to keep in mind that the general principles of LBT are more important than getting specific details right. If we understand both teaching and therapy as processes which confer greater internal degrees of freedom to children, we cannot start from a rigid, fixed position. At the same time, if conditions are too variable, there is not enough stability and structure to create a "holding environment," which is a term used by Donald Winnicott to describe the parent-child relationship and applied it to the facilitative process of therapy (Winnicott, 1965). Creating a safe and secure environment for children to play and interact with each needs to be predictable and stable—especially for children who tend to be anxious and easily distracted by events in the environment—but not rigid or subject to adult-led, "top-down" authoritarian decision-making. Creating a stable and secure holding environment while also being flexible enough to accommodate internal and external changes, and allow for innovation and creativity, are characteristics of any sustainable system, including ecosystems and sociocultural systems.

Some guidelines are straightforward and have been established through years of trial and error by many therapy groups in a range of countries and cultural settings. The usual timeframe for LBT sessions is ninety minutes, with about fifteen minutes of transition time on either side of an hour of active group therapy time. It is not advisable to schedule much less than this time since the other variable parameters will also be affected, such as the number of children in the group, the types and duration of activities, and the ability of the group members to both engage in a construction play activity and spend some time on maintaining the room and the materials. The establishment of interpersonal connections for the participants and being able to work through interpersonal conflicts, discuss future projects, and review the roles and levels of the group members are time-dependent processes.

The group sessions do need a time limit, though, and while some group members—especially more socially mature and self-controlled members—might want to have longer sessions, many of their peers will not be able to tolerate the duration of task focus or sustain their self-discipline (self-monitoring and self-management executive functioning) for more than the basic ninety minutes. The longer duration of groups will also create problems for families and their commitments, or for schools, clinics, and other settings which each have their own schedules of other activities. Keep in mind that a LEGO Club group operates as a system within the context of other physical and sociocultural systems and must collaborate with them.

In that regard, the physical space used for LEGO Club can vary, and so do related variables such as the waiting area, public transportation, parking, accessibility, building common areas, elevators, and restrooms. These variables need to have realistic and sustainable parameters and are often overlooked by therapists or educators who are setting up a group for the first time. In a school or hospital setting, most of these variables will be fixed already or determined administratively. In outpatient clinical settings, much more is open and variable. For instance, setting the time for a group on a weekly basis when the building has a lot of other users can result in problems with parking and common area use. This inevitably results in families arriving late or not at all.

Families are less likely to be able to cope with the additional stress of getting to a group session if they are required to negotiate rush-hour traffic, especially if the site for the group is in a densely urban area. It is invariably the case that participants will have siblings and parents who may not have typical levels of resilience or stress tolerance for sociocultural challenges like getting to places on time, occupying a waiting room for ninety minutes, and accessing a public building and its facilities without leaving behind a trail of physical evidence of their activities. The level of excitement just before and after a group session—with the combined mutual influence of the group members and their friends and family—and the inevitable presence of discarded clothing, toys, electronic devices, food and food containers, and bodily fluids will be a challenge for the therapist and their staff, as well as for many of the group members and their families who may struggle to cope with that environment.

The waiting area should be large enough and have adequate furniture and play materials to accommodate the group members and their families. Anticipate they may arrive early, and often bearing snacks and other materials, and then stay late—either in the waiting room, in the common building areas, or in the parking lot. The waiting area will be loud, and there should be consideration given to keeping that sound from intruding into the playroom itself. The food and play materials should also be kept out of the playroom. This includes LEGO projects which group members may have brought from home, unless there has been an explicit exception made for a given project. The group members should be encouraged to share photos or video images of their own projects, and not bring the LEGO constructions themselves to the group session.

Bringing LEGO from home can lead to confusion about ownership, hard feelings if someone's work is disassembled in some way, or if pieces of it go missing. If there are LEGO materials in the waiting area, make sure they are assigned to that space, and are not taken back and forth between the playroom and the waiting area. It also can negatively affect the sense that the group is a club which has its own materials, members, space, and identity. The LEGO materials in the playroom (or LEGO room), just like the participants themselves, are part of that system, and for the sake of the identity of the group, the LEGO Club needs to be identifiable as such. It is not just a place where some children play with LEGO. It is *the* place where *these* children belong to *this* LEGO Club which happens as *this* time. Without that identity as a group, the synergistic emergent benefits of group membership are lost for the individual participants.

It can be more difficult in school, residential, or hospital settings to get the various elements of a LEGO Club to work together to create the positive experience of interpersonal synergy, group membership, and collaborative accomplishment and shared values. To some extent this is because the group is operating as a subsystem within another system, like a niche within an ecosystem. The group is also temporary, and the group members may change over time, as well as other variables such as the location and the materials. Ideally, having an assigned space just for LBT provides a clear physical representation of the LEGO Club's identity. Children get the sense that this is a LEGO Club immediately when they enter the room, and that physical environment maintains the stability of a specific group's identity over time and across other challenges such as group members coming and going, breaks for holidays, building renovations, and COVID-19 lockdowns.

In addition to the LEGO materials themselves, it can be helpful to have other reminders of the group's identity such as having photos and LEGO posters on the walls, or by having group members share about their experiences and projects on social media. It has become more common for group members to be involved in using media to capture their LEGO projects including digital photos and stop-motion videos which can be shared on group websites or social media sites. This brings up the whole topic of privacy and confidentiality, which varies depending on the context and the relationship between the therapist and their agency and the children, families, and other organizations like libraries, schools, residential facilities, and hospitals which host the groups. These are details that need to be arranged in advance, just like accessibility, furniture, transportation, parking, waiting room space and maintenance, the LEGO materials themselves, etc.

Confidentiality and information sharing among group members, their families, and the agencies and organizations involved will be much different if the group is hosted by a university counseling center, residential treatment facility, children's hospital, a private outpatient clinic, a private school, public school, public library, or a family home. LEGO Club groups have physical, social, cultural, and personal information variables, as well as legal ones. Do not neglect to consider the professional, facility, and organizational liability policies and procedures for risk management and crisis intervention. These issues also apply to protected health information, personal and identity information, and the safety and well-being of the participants and their families. Luckily, for most LBT participants and their families, setting clear parameters for safety and risk management variables is usually experienced in a positive way. Just as the participants usually enjoy participating in setting up and following the LEGO Club rules, their parents are usually reassured by having lots of paperwork and notices about policies and procedures.

Setting up and maintaining a professionally responsible group therapy or social development group can be daunting for some paraprofessional or non-professional individuals who are interested in setting up and running LEGO Club groups. That is for a reason: offering to be helpful to children and their families who are not in your own social circle is a professional, fiduciary commitment which should not be undertaken lightly. Neurodiversity is valuable to society and our species and should be nurtured and supported, not "intervened" with or "treated," like a disease. At the same time, children and their families who have neurodiverse qualities are going to adapt to physical and sociocultural challenges in diverse ways. There is a significant risk of doing harm or creating potentially long-lasting negative effects for children if those who offer to help them also do not fully understand their needs. This is the main issue that was described in my previous book (LeGoff, 2023) about ABA services. Individuals who want to host and facilitate LEGO Club groups need to view it as a professional service and as a fiduciary commitment, which includes having adequate training, experience, and knowledge about child development, family systems, education, learning, and psychopathology. While being autistic is not necessarily a mental disorder (despite being classified as one in the official diagnostic nomenclatures), that does not preclude participants or their family members from having clinically significant mental health challenges.

One of the challenges for LBT discussed further below is the over-diagnosis of autistic conditions, which often results in children being referred for services like LBT (or ABA) who have non-autistic conditions. Differentiating various forms of mental health problems in neurodevelopmental populations is one of the ongoing challenges for which educators and behavior analysts are not typically adequately trained, or qualified. For those therapists who are not qualified mental health providers, ensuring that group members have appropriate access to those services and have had adequate developmental, diagnostic, cognitive, and social evaluations is important. While LBT does not need to be administered by highly trained child psychologists or psychiatrists, those engaging in LBT should have some professional level of training, recognize their own professional limitations, and have access to and utilize additional professional supports when needed.

Participants as members. One of the most important outcomes of LBT is the participants' beneficial experience of identifying with others, being part of both interpersonal and group synergy in collaborative problem solving, shared tasks, and shared creative accomplishments. These experiences also include the formation of peer attachments, which are not feigned, symbolic, or temporary: group members and their families can establish longstanding, meaningful relationships with each other. There are important benefits of social influence and support for group members in many other sociocultural systems, like schools, universities, workplaces, sports and other activities, and communities. For the participants, the LEGO Club may be an introduction to the unforeseen power of sociocultural systems, and it can itself be a powerful influence in their lives.

This is a much different perspective on therapeutic services than is offered by either the medical model "doctor-patient" relationship, or the ABA-based "experimenter-subject," relationship. Neither of these approaches recognize that children are not passive recipients of treatment but are active participants in sociocultural systems. Children are valued by society because they contribute to as well as benefitting from these sociocultural systems, including families, communities, schools, and healthcare systems. Unlike clinical trials for medications or the experimental trials used in ABA interventions, LBT emphasizes the central role of the participants in the developmental process which includes developmentally relevant therapeutic experiences. Just as child development is not based on the emergence of the child's genetic potential alone, or on the influence of a child's environment alone, education and therapy cannot be focused on one or the other but on both and their relationship.

That is why LEGO Club groups emphasize the role of the group members in making decisions for themselves about how they want their group to function as well as on its goals. While the therapist necessarily engages in setting up and maintaining the structure and boundaries of the group, including arranging for funding and meeting the requirements of the agencies and institutions involved, what happens in the LEGO Club system—that is, during the LBT session—should be as much up to the members themselves as possible. During that time, the therapist oversees the group members' safety, but in most situations, they should be in an advisory role to the members who are ultimately responsible for the decisions of the group. At times, the therapist will function as another member of the group and should not assert more authority than any other member would take. Groups' activities and decision-making processes should reflect the norms of their culture. In most modern cultures, which involves democratic decision-making, but including the influence of traditions such as hierarchies based on experience and knowledge, and agreements to allow some group members to take on leadership roles at least temporarily.

During typical LEGO Club groups, the members can decide to led one or two members take the lead on a project, but that is a favor being offered by the other group members for which they can expect some reciprocity or *quid pro quo*. These exchanges of value are a natural part of all human cultures going back to the earliest times of human social group formation. Forming alliances, offering expert input, advice, or skill, and exchanging favors imply that there is some recognized common value involved in those activities. In the case of the LEGO Club, that common value is the shared accomplishment and creativity of the LEGO projects: No one is paid or takes anything away from the group other than the value of being held in esteem by their peers for their contributions. This is also reflected in the value that is subsequently shared by group members with their parents, siblings, friends, and classmates. LEGO Club participants experience being valued by others for having participated as a member of a group which has achieved something valuable which is relevant to their culture (LEGO building is a culturally relevant achievement). For many children, these developmentally important experiences arise from being part of a family, being on a sports team, or joining a youth organization or club, but for children who may not have the level of social motivation to participate in those activities, LEGO Club provides that experience in a personally meaningful way.

Choosing activities and creating a collection. As group members, the LEGO Club participants may naturally want to choose the materials and set up of the room, its furniture, display items, and shelving. That is more easily done if the room is assigned to only one group of children, of course, and that is rarely the case. The more likely scenarios involve several groups of children sharing the space and the materials with other children and other activities. As much as possible, it is important for the therapist to maintain a sense of continuity and a sense of boundary around the LEGO Club's system by being consistent with the physical setting, the timeframe, and the materials available. Even in the situation in which group members are brought together in a generic setting like a therapy or counseling room in a school for one period per week and there are no materials left on display or stored in the room, the therapist can still ensure that the room is set up more or less the same way each week, and that the group members have input to and influence over what materials will become the focus of each group session.

Keeping photos on in an album, or on an electronic device (e.g., camera, phone, or tablet) or uploading them onto a group website are good strategies for supporting a sense of continuity and identity for the group. Maintaining the same set of participants is also important, and group members should be allowed to become familiar with each other and establish a sense of group identity and alliance with other group members across multiple sessions. Using photos of the children themselves along with images of their projects is helpful, although of course, images of the participants will need to be kept confidential more carefully than images of the group projects. These images are reminders to the participants about their competencies and contributions to the group, and a reminder of the synergistic group identity, the LEGO Club, which is more than the sum of its parts (the participants themselves).

The emergent and synergistic quality of group problem-solving and collaborations, as described by Koslowski, *et al*, and Curseu, *et al*, in adult workgroups, also applies to the improved efficiency and creative capacity of LEGO Club groups. It is important for group members to experience this benefit so that they understand its value and are willing to participate in similar situations when given the opportunity in their communities, schools, higher education, and the workplace.

Sorting, organizing, and maintaining materials. From the beginning of a child's involvement in LEGO Club, it is important for them to recognize the value of their contributions to the group not just through LEGO-building activities but through maintaining the integrity of the group's functions and materials. Being committed to a system like a family, sports team, club, or business is expressed in many ways other than fulfilling the basic duties of a group member. Being loyal and supportive towards a sociocultural system is a reciprocally beneficial relationship which, as noted above, also has an element of additional benefit: the emergence of synergistic outcomes. The contributions are made in collaborative ways which improve the overall effectiveness and efficiency of individual efforts, which are experienced in increased value of those efforts.

LEGO materials are an ideal concrete demonstration for the synergistic return-on-investment: LEGO fans (and even those not so familiar with LEGO) appreciate the value of both diligent effort and creativity in the outcome of the sets, freestyle creations, and the stop-motion films produced by group collaborations. Those outcomes are much more achievable and manageable when there are several contributors in different roles collaborating, since the outcomes take much less time to achieve, and there is a sharing of innovative or creative ideas which lead to a greater variety of imaginative projects. Individual projects taken on by individual Club participants will inevitably have a narrower range of ideas and methods of self-expression, as well as a much slower production rate. LEGO materials are quite predictable and can be assessed objectively in terms of the number pieces, and the time commitment, and can also be assessed in subjective ways in terms of their aesthetics, originality, engineering, and design integrity. The LEGO materials themselves, however, also require extensive and diligent maintenance to be accessible for these group projects.

The maintaining of the LEGO therapy room and the LEGO materials will vary a lot depending on the arrangements made to host the LEGO Club sessions. In the situation where there is an assigned room for LBT groups, multiple groups are typically using the same room and materials, so there is naturally a shared responsibility among the different groups and their members to keep the room neat, the materials organized, and the sets and other equipment such as cameras, lighting, and computers in good working order. Having done it myself, I will offer the advice to be diligent about not allowing a diffusion of responsibility: inevitably that will result in the therapist spending all his or her spare time (and spare cash) keeping the room, the materials, and the equipment in good order. When the therapist takes on those responsibilities themselves, that also detracts from the amount of time, effort, and ingenuity that is contributed to, or invested in, the LEGO Club. Contributing their time and efforts to the Club is part of the therapeutic process for all the groups, even those younger group members who may have limited skills and attention span. In the younger groups, the members can still contribute to the Club by doing simple disassembly, sorting, and matching tasks.

One of the ways that group members can contribute (without their parents incurring a financial burden) is to clean, sort, and organize donations of used LEGO. A cost-effective and efficient way for any newer groups to increase their LEGO collection is to advertise to local schools or community resources for donations of used LEGO that is no longer being used at home or in classrooms, etc. Donated LEGO materials can vary a lot in terms of their condition, age, and value of the bricks in terms of being useful for freestyle creations or set restoration. It is not uncommon for LEGO Club prized sets to have bricks missing. This is often a source of stress for the group members, especially if there are missing mini-figs, animals, or other prized pieces (e.g., helmets, weapons, hairpieces, clothing items). Prized pieces like that are sometimes found at the bottom of box of dusty LEGO mixed with candy wrappers, crayons, discarded bandages, rubber bands, and other odd bits and pieces.

Sorting through donated LEGO is usually the first step in the recycling process, and it also involves distinguishing LEGO-brand bricks from knock-offs. Historically, the LEGO Clubs that I have been involved with were true devotees and did not make use of non-LEGO imitations. The LEGO copyright for the interlocking brick system was filed initially in Denmark in 1958 (internationally in 1961), and those copyrights began expiring in the 2000's. Despite legal attempts by LEGO Corporation to maintain their patent rights on their brick design, by 2011, their patents had all but disappeared, and the toy manufacturer was required to seek continued product innovation and development rather than to continue to restrict other manufacturers from copying and selling their designs. Personally, from my own ethical perspective, LEGO as a cultural contribution should have been protected by the courts. The imitators do not have the same level of quality, in my view, from the plastic itself to the quality of engineering in the designs and their building instructions. LEGO itself has a brand identity because of its history which is a synergistic emergence, like so many other culturally relevant products. The decision to be exclusive to LEGO-brand LEGO or not I will leave to the reader, but I wanted to be clear: even though I have no relationship with LEGO Corporation of any kind and have never been given gifts or even a discount on LEGO products, I am still brand loyal, which reflects the value I attribute to the cultural contributions that LEGO has made.

Both child and adult LEGO fans are familiar with the amount of labor involved in keeping track of specific set pieces as well as in sorting bricks from random collections into specific bins or trays. This is one of the most important "helper," activities described below, but it is also a whole-group activity. Without some level of organization and sorting of random bricks, and diligently maintaining set bricks, both set-integrity and creative freestyle building is severely hampered. Although it may take hours to sort through bins and to sort them—including arranging the containers and bins for keeping them sorted and organized—the investment of that effort is well worth the investment when it comes to creating and building. LEGO bricks can be put through a dishwasher (in a mesh bag), but they then need to be sorted and organized into bins. The bins may need to be labeled, and organized, often using plastic drawers on wheels, and using large cafeteria trays to hold parts while they are being sorted or while under construction.

Even in situations where the LEGO room is shared with other activities or needs to be portable, the LEGO materials need to be organized and contained in some way. That not only allows the group members to work on their organizational and critical thinking skills, but it also reflects the sorts of activities that are valuable in any sociocultural system: maintaining the homeostasis of the system. While they are not often considered highly valued or glamorous roles, all of us intuitively assign a sense of value to others in our families, businesses, clubs, associations, and teams who do the chores: making the coffee, sorting and assigned the mail and other communications, creating and administering budgets, re-stocking the common areas with tissues, flowers, candy, hand-sanitizer, and air freshener, putting hand towels and toilet tissue in the restrooms, buying birthday cards and getting them signed, or ordering a cake for a special occasion, organizing fund-raisers, etc.

Those seemingly unappreciated and anonymous tasks are shared by us all, and they are a common part of what makes life in our communities and workplaces seem more humane and worthwhile. We do not ask LEGO Club members to do those tasks, but there are many similar ones which need to be accomplished in LEGO Club like cleaning and sorting used bricks, looking for missing pieces, or re-sorting jumbled junk drawers of parts. Caring about each other and about the group is part of being a group member, and so it is an important part of learning how to participate in sociocultural systems by being in the LEGO Club.

The "Rules of Cool"—implicit social norms. As was described in the previous chapter, the LEGO Club has some explicit rules—preferably developed and implemented by the group members themselves—as well implicit rules. The explicit rules are necessary for the maintaining the structure of the group as a sociocultural system within the context of other responsibilities of the professionals hosting the group, the parents, the building management, or the school administration. These are externally oriented rules and reflect the influence of other systems which impose restrictions and social norms in exchange for civil rights and protections. The Rules of Cool relate to codes of conduct that are directed internally towards the other members of the group and reflect the value that group members give to each other. Being valued and feeling valued by others is a core part of how LEGO Club benefits its participants. That value, however, does not have a common label or description, despite being central to all sociocultural systems.

The value that individuals who participate in sociocultural systems have towards each other is not just a human value since it is essentially the same as that which we hold towards other species, or specific members of other species with whom we have relationships, like our pets, service animals, or farm animals. We value them and each other as living beings. This inherent value of living organisms is a topic that will be described in another book, but for now it is enough to say that it derives from the recognition the living organisms are unique, both because of their genetic makeup and their lived experiences, and contribute to the perpetuation of life as a system on this planet. The reader is directed to the works of Peter Corning for an in-depth discussion of the scientific rationale for thinking about life and evolution as a collaborative system (Corning, 2022; 2005) rather than being a competitive one. In this view, the goal of life for all species, including homo sapiens, is not to become the dominant species on the planet, but to support the adaptability of life as a system. Participating creatively in life as a system implies that we value each other and that we value each other's collaborative, creative, and diverse contributions. That is the spirit and philosophy of LEGO Club: sharing the achievement of a sustainable, creative, and adaptable system.

The general principle underlying adaptable participation in life is the same as that underlying the Rules of Cool which guide interpersonal interactions in LEGO Club: sharing, balancing, and growing degrees of freedom. A degree of freedom in life or in LEGO Club is pretty much the same as what it is in physics, statistics, and physiology: an undetermined or unfixed variable. If a variable is determined or fixed, whether it is internal to an individual or external and part of their environment, it is not understood. While we do not need to fully understand how a system works to exert influence over it, to the extent that we get to choose the values of a variable, we have internalized those degrees of freedom because the value for them is determined by our internal processes. Some internal degrees of freedom are built into our genetic makeup and physiology so that infants can learn to perceive the world around them and begin to organize their movements in relation to the physical and social world that they sense and perceive. The control over organized, skillful movement is a process that involves both the unfolding of the genetically designed skeletal, muscular, sensory-perceptual, and neurological systems of our bodies in interaction with what Winnicott called the facilitating environment.

What children are demonstrating as they develop is the internalization of the degrees of freedom of the events both within and outside of them. Some events we control unconsciously and automatically, while others require considerable sustained attention, effort, and skill, but in both cases, we are never fully in control of any event: we participate in it. It was the American poet Robert Frost who was quoted as saying about freedom, "I guess one way of putting it would be that you have freedom when you're easy in your harness." Being one part of the whole system of life does not mean that we are not free, or that we can be completely free. It means that we have some capacity to freely choose what to do, or at least, what to think or feel. The difference between living organisms and inert matter is ultimately that simple: organisms can choose how to be. With that freedom, however, comes the responsibility to ensure that our actions are consistent with the system, life, which has allowed us that freedom. In other words, we must always be aware of our harness, which is the context in which we have freedom, which is the system of life in which we participate.

The Rules of Cool reflect existing interpersonal values and ideals which support individuals to maintain their own internalized degrees of freedom, including their genetic individuality and unique life-experiences, while respecting that of those around them. Even more importantly, though, being able to participate creatively in a sociocultural system (or an ecosystem), means that individuals can collaborate or to generate synergistic, emergent outcomes. All members of the LEGO Club need to learn through in-the-moment experiences how to share their interests, skills, experience, and creativity, while at the same time, flexibly accommodating those of their fellow members. Many individuals can participate in sociocultural systems and maximize their own degrees of freedom and those of the systems in which they participate from birth: they naturally develop those powers. These are socially influential people who become leaders and powerful members of society. All members of society, however, share some of that power because we all have some freedom to choose how we will participate and thereby contribute value.

What LEGO Club members intuitively recognize as "cool," is the growth of both individual and group power that results from synergistic collaboration. To some extent that involves direct interpersonal communication and interaction, but it also involves indirect contributions to the emergent degrees of freedom of the group as whole. Individual group members collaborate with each other, but the group as a whole is responsible for its creative output, and its persistence as a group. The LEGO Club in that sense is a microcosm of other sociocultural systems, which are themselves microcosms of larger systems such as societies or ecosystems. In ethological terms, LEGO Club is like a niche, but it is supported in part by a host organism (the group leader or therapist), and it is unusual in that it is temporary and sporadic (it comes to life once a week at a given time). In the minds of the group members, though, or on social media, the LEGO Club is continuous. As many former LEGO Club members and therapists can also attest, it continues to exist in their minds for years afterwards.

Activities and relationships outside of the LEGO Club. Like many other complex and growing organic systems, LEGO Club typically begins with an intense focus on its own operations and dynamics. Slowly over time, the group members will naturally expand their fields of operation to include other individuals and systems. This process does not need much facilitation, in my experience, but unfolds naturally like the group activities themselves, and the main role of the therapist or facilitator is to not interfere. It is not as simple as that, however, since there may be some influences which are potentially harmful or which would interfere with the operation and homeostasis of the LEGO Club if introduced too early, or in ways that interfere with the bonding and activities that sustain the group. This includes the group members inviting friends or siblings to participate, having parents invited in to view the ongoing process, group members visiting other LEGO Clubs, or having a group member's family, school, or other group (e.g., church group or Boy Scouts) sponsor an activity or host a session.

Inviting outside social influences or materials is like having food in the LEGO Club: it can be fine if the group members are prepared to control those degrees of freedom. Uncontrolled variability in sociocultural settings is the underlying problem that group members are struggling with. Disciplining group members by giving them a "time-out," suspending them for a certain number of sessions, or expelling them outright, is one dramatic example of how unregulated degrees of freedom introduce an unacceptable level of stress. Children with autistic conditions typically appreciate and benefit from reductions in undetermined sociocultural degrees of freedom because, whether they are consciously aware of it or not, they do not have internal degrees of freedom to allow them to predict and control those systems. That is also why they do not do well in social or educational settings which have many people: the underdetermined degrees of freedom in those systems increase exponentially with the number of individuals and their interactions with each other.

Introducing an unknown variable, such as how a fellow group member will experience being excluded from the group—an experience they themselves are horrified to imagine—needs to be considered in the context of the internally moderated or determined degrees of freedom of the individuals in the group, as well as those that are part of the established group system. If group members have established rules and routines, even if they do not have many sociocultural degrees of freedom internalized individually, the group will be more tolerant of adaptive challenges. Stress tolerance, in that sense, whether it is of an individual or a system, reflects the internal degrees of freedom which allow that individual or system to adapt to environmental challenges. As Winnicott originally described, the facilitating environment of a parent, or any other supportive setting, such as a therapeutic or educational one, needs to titrate environmental challenges. In the case of LEGO Club, that means ensuring that the group members have an established routine and have had adequate experience of the other members and group dynamics as whole for both the individuals and the group to be stable enough to tolerate change while maintaining their internal order, as well as having enough expertise or skill in managing the degrees of freedom of that setting to be flexible and creative.

Bernstein (1948/1996) provided an excellent description of the process by which individuals acquire skills by initially freezing and then freeing degrees of freedom of a complex movement. What that involves is observable in most children and adults as they learn a new motor skill: they simplify the action by holding certain variables of movement—joints or whole-body parts—in a stable position so they can focus more attention and control on others. Novices in acquiring a complex skilled movement are sometimes encouraged by mentors or coaches in their scaffolding attempts to limit the overall complex activity to just specific components of it. Holding certain degrees of freedom of a complex system—such as a complex movement—allows the internal prediction and control of a more limited number of degrees of freedom, and once those are accomplished by the motor system, additional degrees of freedom can be added. That is how any skilled movement changes over time from being more limited and stiffer, or frozen, to being more fluid, creative and adaptable while still maintaining a high level of skilled execution over time.

That same principle of limiting or freezing degrees of freedom—undetermined variables—at first to acquire some increased level of skill before adding variables to the system applies to any sociocultural system. Adding variability to a system before that system has the internal ability to predict and control those degrees of freedom will result in a natural experience of being overwhelmed and distressed, which may elicit regression. Synergy can be understood as from a systems perspective as an organization of diverse elements whose relationship and interaction results in emergent outcomes, or new degrees of freedom. Synergy is creative in the sense that the systems involved in synergistic processes create events or exchanges of energy and information reflecting degrees of freedom (variability of events) which previously did not exist. This is just as applicable to systems like a family or a classroom as it is to a society or to an individual child. Antergy refers to the inverse of synergy such that diverse elements of a system stop operating freely, becoming fixed, or cease to exist, resulting in a loss of degrees of freedom for that system.

Progression and regression in development: Synergy and antergy. In the context of child development, internal synergy involves a child's internal physiological and mental system (a self-system) operating in ways which are creative and result in novel internal degrees of freedom, such as coming up with new ideas or having insights, which is not the same as simply learning information that is made available. Knowing information is additive, but understanding information, which involves emergent insights about the information, is synergistic. External synergy in the physical and sociocultural environment is also involved in child development, but the child is a participant in systems outside of themselves and they contribute to the determination of the degrees of freedom of those systems as well as within themselves. In that sense, Vygotsky's ZPD and Bruner's scaffolding involve children participating in systems of energy exchange and information which are larger and more complex than themselves, and by doing so, they adapt by internalizing knowledge and understanding that is relevant to their participation in those systems. That is synergistic growth and development.

Play and learning are developmentally important because they involve synergy and creativity which lead to increased levels of internal degrees of freedom which improve adaptability. For children who are growing in their adaptive capacity, as opposed to many adults who are holding steady at a given level of functioning, or possibly in slow decline (me included), it is not expected or normal for them to stall or to stop progressing in the expansion of the internal degrees of freedom of their self-system. That does not mean that a child would stop learning, but they may not continue to process what they learn in synergistic ways; they stop having insights and understanding what they are learning, or they stop developing skills that are commensurate with their increased physical size and strength.

Latash (2021) outlined the ways in which internally controlling the degrees of freedom of a skilled purposeful movement is like the process of understanding (having a higher-order cognitive model) information. In that sense a motor skill is a systematic operation like understanding; it requires a synergistic emergence, or higher-order cognitive model of the degrees of freedom of that complex physical or cognitive event. When we can stop simply operating within the physical, sociocultural, or informational system and can have insights about that system, we are able to be creative and play with it. That is how we can improve and play with both our actions (as in a game or a sport, or in executing a work of art or playing a musical instrument) and our ideas (having insights, daydreaming, brainstorming). Play is the operative dynamic in both mental creativity and creative actions, and it is an inherently synergistic process.

When a child regresses, they are not just stalling in their progression or increasing their capacity to participate in the determination of degrees of freedom inside and outside of themselves; they lose the capacity to participate in both internal and external degrees of freedom. When we lose information, like forgetting something, that is not a developmental regression because we still have the adaptive capacity to regain that information and we still retain the insight about how to use that information. Similarly, if we get rusty or unaccustomed to a given skill—we have not played golf or tennis or ridden a bicycle in a while—our control of the degrees of freedom for that complex action will not have regressed necessarily. We can quickly recover that competency so that is not a developmental regression. Our internal self-system still includes those degrees of freedom. If we completely forget how to do something, or if we are so intimidated by an activity, we refuse to participate at all, that is a functional regression. In those situations, we choose not to participate, or in some cases, our internal and external systems are restricting us from participating in those systems. When an individual does not participate in a system, they lose the degrees of that system from their self-system, and simultaneously, that system loses the degrees of freedom—the internal, unique, creative processes—of that individual. The various elements of internal and external systems which result in a loss of adaptive capacity for both individuals and the systems in which they participate, is antergy. Developmental regression, as opposed to developmental halts or stalling, or simply maturation, results from antergistic operations. Some types of antergy are mild and may be normal such as occur with aging, although many would say that aging involves an increased level of insight (wisdom) and the amount of loss of access to new information is more than made up for by that level of understanding. Developmental regression is not normal in children and young adults, however, and usually reflects antergistic or pathological processes, whether that is due to a physical illness or maladaptive sociocultural processes. In the case of autistic conditions, there is no reason to expect children not to show persistent development and growth, even if that development may be atypical from a sociocultural perspective. Children, like all living organisms, typically grow in their adaptive capacity as their bodies and brains mature, and as they learn through experience. As noted above, what causes regression is not usually a single factor or event, but antergistic dynamic among multiple factors which result in them being excluded from participation in their relevant systems. In the case of autistic children, the most common regressive influence is anxiety, followed by systematic exclusion.

Anxiety and stress are the most common long term negative life experiences which inhibit child and young adult development for autistic individuals. The conditions which result in those experiences are predictably due to difficulties understanding and participating in sociocultural systems, which can result in chronic maladaptive outcomes in terms of inadequate social support, low income, and over-dependence on parents or other family members. For younger children, anxiety and stress are more commonly involved in social isolation, irritability and anger, diminished learning, and increased levels of rigid, repetitive maladaptive actions. The insistence on sameness and obsessive-compulsive tendencies observed in autistic children are best understood as predictable consequences of feeling helpless and unable to understand how to participate in the sociocultural systems around them and are characteristic of any child who experiences those sorts of life conditions.

Children who feel overwhelmed and unable to cope with the challenges in their environment experience what clinicians refer to as trauma, and they often regress in ways that are like how autistic children response to similar experiences (Dozio, *et al*, 2020; Robinson-Drummer, *et al*, 2019; Fuld, 2018; Arsenio, *et al*, 2009; McDonald, *et al*, 2008). The types of intervention strategies for children who have experienced psychological trauma are also like that which is indicated for overcoming social avoidance and anxiety responses in children with autism (Humble, *et al*, 2018). This is not to imply that being autistic is the result of psychological trauma or stressful social experiences. The evidence does suggest, however, that being autistic increases children's exposure to overwhelming or traumatically stressful events which lead to increased experiences of helplessness and mistrust of others which can exacerbate difficulties with social development and lead to clinically significant and chronic problems with social anxiety, social avoidance, and socially mediated learning. Just as importantly, not feeling safe and secure in typical learning environments like the classroom or playground can inhibit play. Inhibition of play is itself also a potential contributor to stalls or regressions in the development of motor, cognitive, language, and social skills (Ha, 2022; Koeners & Francis, 2020; Muentener, Herrig & Schulz, 2018; Nijhof, *et al*, 2018; Liu, *et al*, 2017; Kirkham, Stuart & Kidd, 2013; Wang & Aamodt, 2012; LaFreniere, 2011; Hughes, 2010; Ginsburg, *et al*, 2007; Lewis, et al, 2000).

While many researchers have emphasized the importance of allowing children to play as part of their educational experiences and curricula (Whitebread, *et al*, 2017; Pelligrini, 2009; Pellegrini & Smith, 2008, 1998), others have emphasized the lifelong importance of play in human health, creativity, socialization, and vocational success (Singha, *et al*, 2020; Siviy, 2016; Tsai, 2012; Pellis & Pellis, 2009), including the founders of the constructivist movement in education and child development, Jean Piaget (1962b), Lev Vygotsky (1967), and Jerome Bruner (1986; 1973). An extensive and growing body of literature has demonstrated that play is not a learned behavior (c.f., LeGoff, 2023, for further discussion), and in fact it occurs spontaneously as an important feature of skill acquisition and socially mediated learning in many other species (Vanderschuren, Achterburg & Trezza, 2016; Siviy & Panskepp, 2011; Smith, 2006). Play is strongly associated with increased levels of cognitive, communication, and social functioning as well as creativity and adaptability not only in children but across species (Wah, 2020).

CHAPTER 6

ROLES, TASKS, AND LEVELS IN LEGO-BASED THERAPY

Different roles in synergistic systems. As Mark Latash has described in literate and scientific detail (Latash, 2008), the principles of synergy operate in systems in which there are elements which contribute in diverse ways to a common outcome or goal. This has also been described in equally refined and detailed ways by Peter Corning (2018). David Araujo and Keith Davids have also described similar operational dynamics extensively in the field of sports psychology (Araujo & Davids, 2106; 2011). Each of these writers come from different scientific backgrounds and contexts, but they describe similar phenomena and identify the same necessary characteristics of synergy in homeostatic systems. In the simplest terms, for a group of diverse elements to form a system that is potentially self-sustaining, it must have a boundary, as was discussed above, and it must have various components which perform different functions or roles. The functions of the components within the system need to be both complementary and collaborative, as well as being able to sustain the system and its growth through environmental challenges. The internal diversity and organization of components of a homeostatic system are also necessarily stable in some way, and able to maintain their integrity and identity.

In the LEGO Club and LBT, the idea of creative synergy was not an explicit goal but was identified by me as a necessity from the outset. If I wanted the children I was working with to learn how to work together, they would need to be motivated in a way to do that, and that would require me to provide a safe and stable setting for that to happen (therapy sessions in a play room) and to get them to share a common task (LEGO building) with different, complementary roles (part-supplier, builder, and engineer). That initial and simple form of interpersonal synergy immediately had the effect that I had hoped it would: both boys and I realized we were on to something; we could build LEGO creations much faster and with more creativity if we maintained different roles and responsibilities and contributed our own unique ideas and skills towards a common goal. We became the LEGO version of Andre Dumas' three musketeers, "One for all, and all for one!"

Hierarchies and Communication in systems and LEGO Club. The different roles which participants assume in the group vary informally based on individual and group activities determined by the tasks a group member is working on for a group project. There should not be any individual activities which do not involve the group, unless they are done outside of the group sessions. The roles are also affected by the types of LEGO-based activities, which tend to become more elaborate over time in terms of the project itself and the skills involved in completing them, and the group members themselves are also able to participate in higher levels of task complexity as well as authority in the group's chain of command or decision-making hierarchy.

Like the principle of diversity of roles in adaptable systems, hierarchical organization is another central feature of synergistic systems including individual organisms (Latash, 2008; Bernstein, 1947/2020). Both the diversity of roles and the necessity for levels in the decision-making process are characteristic of adaptive systems, and they necessitate some form of ongoing internal communication—feedback loops—which are central to homeostatic operations (task management) as well as for adaptive innovation and creativity. Successful families, classrooms, teams, businesses, communities, and societies, utilize both hierarchical levels and communication within and between levels (Brody, 1973; Laszlo, 1972a & b). The roles and activities within the level hierarchy in LEGO Club is typical of many other systems in that it is more flexible for individuals at higher levels than for those at lower levels. This is a natural outcome of the fact that group members are required to demonstrate to their peers in the group that they have acquired the skills (internalized degrees of freedom of the relevant systems) for a given level before they can take on responsibilities which are assigned to the next level. These levels are described in detail in the next chapter.

Individual group members demonstrate acquisition of a hierarchy of skill-sets, from the basic skills of putting sets together (following visual directions, sorting, selecting, and assembling bricks) to directing and managing the completion of large, multi-session projects. The group also demonstrates the capacity to take on more elaborate projects and so their activities go through a series of stages, from set-building to stop-motion filmmaking. As noted above, however, the individual members and the group have some flexibility with respect to their chosen activities once they have internalized the degrees of freedom of those projects. A LEGO Club group which is learning how to operate efficiently in putting sets together or collaborating on freestyle projects is not ready to take on stop-motion filmmaking, but a group which is actively making stop-motion films will still want (and need) to do collaborative set and freestyle constructing.

This is a characteristic of many synergistic systems, although there are typically limits to which higher-level individuals or elements will continue to participate in lower-level activities, or take on lower-level projects, since that is often inefficient, or no longer feasible from an operational point of view. The individual with higher level decision-making and skillset, however, still retains the internal degrees of freedom of the lower-level operations. Orchestra conductors need to understand the degrees of freedom and parameters of expected outcomes for each of the orchestra members. A business owner or executive is more effective when they have internalized the degrees of freedom and parameters of output of each member of their organization, and each unit or division. What is important for the higher level of decision-making is not that they participate in all levels of the system, but that they can effectively and efficiently direct their operations, including making innovative or creative decisions. While most of the activities of a LEGO Club, for example, can occur through individual communication about a specific task (like the daily operations of a business, or the interactions of teammates on the field), for a group to achieve something, there needs to be top-down decision-making, especially if the outcome involves innovative or creative designs.

The LEGO Club activities can accommodate and benefit from diverse skill levels—the participants work their way up the hierarchy of levels as different rates—and in different roles or tasks on different projects, but also from individual differences in abilities, skills, and interests. Although group members are encouraged to work together on common goals, and the group activities emphasize common values and interests, the LEGO Club remains highly flexible and adaptable in terms of the projects themselves. One of the benefits of using LEGO as a play material is that it can accommodate an infinite array of interests or pre-occupations. For children who do not initially identify themselves as a LEGO fan, they will likely have some activity or topic area that is of interest to them which can become the focus of LEGO-based creative activities. It is these individual interests and knowledge bases that contribute to the richness and creative potential of the LEGO Club experience.

This is why the communication about LEGO projects is not left entirely up to the more experienced or more skilled LEGO Club members. Even the group members who are still improving their basic LEGO skills at the helper or builder levels have creative ideas which should be shared with the group and enrich the LEGO Club's creative output. Although some group members may not develop the fine motor or engineering or design capabilities to produce elaborate LEGO creations on their own, they may have good visualization abilities and can communicate verbally or through drawing, or even using gestures or pictures from other media (e.g., images downloaded on a smartphone) to share their creative ideas with the group. Some group members may excel at creating visual or verbal narratives which the group can use to create stop-motion animated films.

The LBT groups have traditionally encouraged members to express themselves and be responsive to input from others using all forms of communication simultaneously. Many group members have advanced language abilities, while others might have weaknesses in this area, but all group members (based on their needs) may struggle with effective social communication. The important point is not to increase verbal communication skills, necessarily—although LEGO Club does seem to help with that—but to improve the motivation and capacity to share ideas and collaborate on mutually beneficial projects. Sharing values for LEGO, for the Club, for each other, and for their collaborative efforts is the emphasis, not just skill development. For the children themselves, they may be eager to get to the higher levels of the group hierarchy, which requires both LEGO-based and interpersonal communication skills, but that motivation is more important than the skills per se, because that is what will improve their sociocultural adaptation outside of the group. Being good with LEGO, and even being able to communicate and collaborate effectively, are of only limited benefit if a child does not experience an increased level of identification with peers and motivation to participate in sociocultural systems outside of the Club, at home, at school, in the community, and eventually, in the workplace. The improvements in interpersonal interaction and communication seem natural and even inevitable, though, once a child begins identifying with others and wanting to collaborate with them, both in the LEGO Club and outside of it.

CHAPTER 7

STAGES OF ACTIVITIES AND THE LEVEL SYSTEM IN LEGO CLUB

As discussed in the previous chapter, LEGO Club members are given the opportunity to participate in collaborative activities through which they experience the benefits of synergistic dynamics. These include the collaboration of individuals filling different, complementary roles who may have differing interests as well as skillsets, as well as being at different levels in the LEGO Club's internal hierarchy of skill development. The activities which group members engage in, and the projects they take on as a group, begin with smaller, structured activities like building small sets, and then gradually increased in size, degree of modification and innovation, and finally, increasingly ambitious freestyle creations. Beyond that level, there are even more complex stop-motion animation projects which require LEGO-based as well as other skills and high levels of interpersonal communication and collaboration. Most of the hierarchical organization of the LEGO Club groups is informal, but there is a formal hierarchy which is the individual group members' level system, which evolved organically over time from the group members' interest in sharing a mutual respect for their own and their fellow group members' skills and achievements.

Set building. The original and what seemed to be the most obvious way to ensure interpersonal communication and collaboration during group therapy sessions was the division of labor process described in the first article on LBT (LeGoff, 2004). Demonstrating competence in three core skills of LEGO set building has continued to today as a sort of traditional right of passage for LEGO Club members. From the outset, since there were originally only two group members and I involved, there has been some tension about adding new group members. A natural result of the synergistic success of the first triad (the two first group members and myself being engineer, builder, and part supplier), was that other children saw evidence that there was LEGO building happening in the playroom and they wanted to participate. In various ways, all forms of play are representational.

Play is made up of symbolic actions within a certain culture or society that involve participation in activities, usually with peers, which require increasing proficiency with culturally relevant adaptive skills: communication and language, interpersonal interaction based on social norms and values, and culturally specific technology (from sticks to computers). LEGO building just happens to be a form of play which is both widely popular in many cultures and societies, and the skills involved have clear relevance to many basic work skills, such as inductive and deductive reasoning, attention to detail, fine motor skills, sustaining mental set, following feedback loops, and problem solving. When the overall process of set or freestyle building is divided into different but complementary roles among different children, there is an initial resistance from the participants since many children are already familiar with LEGO building as an individual activity, but if encouraged to persist with the activity—which is easily done by just not giving them a choice; they either participate with others, or they will be left out of the activity—they quickly experience the synergistic outcomes. Putting LEGO sets together is much more efficient when the task is functionally divided using a horizontal—as opposed to vertical—task analysis and shared collaboratively. That process and format for the activity of LEGO building turns out to be a useful way to approach many other potentially beneficial sociocultural systems.

In addition to understanding the value of synergies between group members in task completion and experiencing the shared identification with others and the value of shared accomplishments, the initial set-building triad experience introduces group members to the idea that sharing an activity does not detract from it, but in fact adds to the value of the activity. Most children have some experiences of feeling initially disappointed about having to share an experience with others, like sharing any preferred item like a toy or a snack with others. Sharing in that sense diminishes the value of the experience. Over time, however, children experience sharing in positive ways, especially when they identify with others such as their parents and siblings, and they resonate empathically with their positive experiences. Sharing a laugh, or a meal, or a game becomes the primary motivator for engaging in fun, rewarding activities. Among typical children, many are born knowing that interpersonal connectedness is the foundation for all other values since they do not experience pleasurable events as satisfying or meaningful unless they are shared.

As was mentioned earlier, for many children in LEGO Club, the initial set-building triad may be their first experience of why other more sociable children have this attitude towards sharing experiences. While many autistic children will understand that it is a norm or a rule that one should play games with other children, share play materials with them, or share their food or other resources with them, they struggle with experiencing that as somehow more pleasurable than doing those activities on their own. It is difficult for them to understand how undertaking a skill-related activity—practicing something or learning about something—can be enhanced through social sharing, or how problem solving, and creativity can be better. "Two heads are better than one," is just a platitude to them. Most children and adults intuitively know that the joy involved in an activity is multiplied by the number of people, not divided by it, but that requires them to see those others as being like themselves, affiliated with them, or somehow part of themselves. Sociable people have an intuitive awareness that their self-system includes the energy, resourcefulness, and joy of other people with whom they identify. If they experience others as "them," and not "us," then that experience of the synergistic benefit of shared experiences is lost. For autistic children, they rarely experience a sense of "us," and almost all social activities involve "them."

For the LEGO Club members, being able to do the basic LEGO tasks of set-building seems to be a symbolic requirement for being a group member above the level of being just a Helper, but they also have an intuitive awareness that those who have gone through the experience of set-building as part of a triad also now understand interpersonal synergy. That seems to be one of the unspoken but obvious elements that carries on throughout the LEGO Club experience: the acknowledgement of social belonging or "like me," experience of the group members for each other. This seems like some type of initiation ritual experience which is common to other types of social groups or clubs and initiates a sense of shared purpose through common experiences. "They," become an "us," by being "like me," because they share an interest and an experience which yields the shared insight that being part of an "us," is much better than just being by oneself. Although there are some who might want to forgo the initial set-building triad experience as part of being in a LEGO Club, it is important to keep in mind that it is not simply a way to demonstrate a member's competence in LEGO set-building, it is an opportunity for them to demonstrate to themselves and to the others that they are in fact a member of the group, one of *us*.

Free style creating and building. To those unfamiliar with LEGO processes, they may not understand the distinction between free-style creating and free-style building—or even between free-style LEGO and set-building—but the differences are relevant and important. Building involves selecting bricks and putting them together, and since virtually all LEGO bricks can be interconnected with any other LEGO brick, putting pieces together can be a random activity. It is a common experience for those who have LEGO materials on hand that putting a few bricks together more or less randomly can result in some surprisingly creative outcomes. We usually start out by sifting through a bin of bricks and almost daydreaming, letting the materials and our fingers interact without much guidance from our higher order cognitive processes.

This is like a process which has been studied extensively in connection with creativity and play in general by the neuroscientist Jonathan Smallwood and his colleagues (Smallwood & Schooler, 2014; Smallwood, 2013; Smallwood & Schooler, 2006). They have found that when we allow our minds to wander, the human brain is adept at noticing and taking advantage of its own complex, semi-random operations. In other words, when we daydream or let our minds wander, part of our brain keeps track of where it is going and uses that meandering as a way of getting new ideas that we might not come up with otherwise. In that sense, building something like a LEGO set, is using an external structure to reduce the degrees of freedom of our internal system (at least temporarily). By doing so, however, we add that rigid, fixed model, like the directions for a set, or a method of putting bricks together, as a construct, or in physiological terms what the neuropsychologist Donald Hebb called cell assemblies (Hebb, 1949). Creating internal functional representations of objects, actions, and relationships based on our experiences of systems of events around us is essentially the process of internalizing degrees of freedom. When we allow part of our brain's cell assemblies to relax their normal associative connections and play together almost randomly, the results can be like looking through a kaleidoscope, looking at clouds going by, or picking out LEGO bricks from a bin: we allow randomness to add diversity and variability to our internal degrees of freedom.

This process of letting our minds wander but keeping track of where it goes has social applications as well. This was the process that was described by Sigmund Freud (1938) and his followers as "free association," which played a central role in the process of psychoanalysis. In that context, the analyst offered the structuring interpretations of the personal, emotional, and unconscious meaning of seemingly random but somehow representational dreams, free associations, and mistakes, which Freud referred to as parapraxes, which were meaning-laden accidents. Smallwood position is that all of us engage in forms of psychoanalysis when we pay attention to our loosely connected thoughts and images. This is also a common theme in various versions of psychic healing, fortune-telling, Tarot-card, or tealeaf reading: the potential of randomness to add power and meaning to otherwise mundane and predictable events. Aside from seeking expert advice on combining random information to enhance creative interpretations of events, many people participate in spontaneous interpersonal creativity in brainstorming sessions, jazz music, or improvisational performances.

Just as improvisation in music starts with changing a few notes and can lead to writing entire jazz compositions, freestyling in LEGO Club starts with just modifying or revising a few bricks in a set and can lead to designing and engineering unique creations. In this sense, some forms of improvisation in LEGO Club are considered innovative, such as using an existing set and building it out of spare LEGO bricks, or modifying a LEGO set for use in a scene or action sequence of a stop-motion film. The integrity of the set design is not changed, but its appearance or function might be improved or altered for a specific purpose. Innovating with LEGO is not the same as creating, but both involve building. Creating with LEGO involves contributing an idea, usually a functional structure or three-dimensional form, which is novel to that LEGO Club. It is difficult to be completely original given that millions of children and adults use LEGO materials creatively every day around the world, but then, human diversity and creativity is truly endless, so some LEGO Club creations will be unique.

It is the process of starting with an idea, then identifying the bricks and their structural organization to achieve the desired outcome, which defines a LEGO freestyle creation, as opposed to an innovation. The group member who comes up with an idea can be credited with that as a LEGO Creator project even if they do not build it themselves. It is considered an even higher level of skill to come up with ideas and convince the other group members to build them. Some LEGO Creators, who are working at the level of LEGO Experts or LEGO Genius, will be temporarily in a leadership role and can ask other group members to both engineer and build a LEGO creation that they have designed, just as an architect might ask engineers and builders to fill in the details on their design of a building. What is important to the LEGO Club, though, is that all the group members participate in various ways in both the conceptualization, engineering, and building of the project, so that it is not just one group member's achievement, but an achievement of the LEGO Club as a whole.

Creating scenes and stop-motion films. As will be described below, there are mutually accepted standards or skills associated with the level system in LEGO Club and those have been determined by the group members, largely based on what is required by the demands of the projects themselves. Although the creative potential of LEGO is endless, the process of starting with an idea, coming up with a design, and then building it out of LEGO bricks involves some physical and material engineering challenges, especially if that idea involves function as well as appearance. For some years, prior to the advent of LEGO still scenes (photographed images of LEGO depicting a scene, like a travel picture, advertisement photo, and action shot or poster from a film) and then stop-motion animated films, complex LEGO creations were the pinnacle of activities in LEGO Club. Many of those creations were designed and engineered to demonstrate the functional capacity of LEGO materials and the ingenuity of the group members in engineering and building them.

Some of the projects undertaken by LEGO Clubs were impressive, such as building very tall towers of bricks, often reaching from the table surface (not the floor, for practical reasons—cleaning staff and other kids moving around in the room) to the ceiling. Designing and engineering a tall tower without it toppling over required a lot of collaborative communication on design strategies and construction time, materials, and focused effort. Some group members proposed creative ideas like creating a LEGO stadium, roller coaster, airport, zoo, or theme park, or they would propose building an entire town or city with multiple buildings. These were the sorts of projects that were the ultimate level of LEGO Club activity which required a group member to take on a leadership role on that project from idea to completion.

By the end of a project like that, most group members would have either failed and would then know what they needed to improve on—usually in their interpersonal skills, organization and task management, or self-management skills, since their LEGO skills were usually at a high level by that point—or they succeeded. Succeeding at a task like that would usually result in the child, their parents, the therapist, and other parties including the LEGO Club and even the member's school staff, that they no longer needed LEGO Club as therapy. By that point, they were usually at or above age-level in terms of being able to effectively participate in sociocultural and educational activities.

In the late 1990's, however, one LEGO Club member asked the other group members if they would help him use LEGO to do a stop-motion film depicting the story of the NASA Apollo 13 moon rocket project. The group member had sold his history teacher at school on the idea of submitting a short, animated film using his Hi8 camcorder instead of a written essay on the subject. The group members agreed to use some of the space exploration themed LEGO sets and then create the other designs that would be needed. The student provided a storyboard and script for the short film, and the group members built the sets, and then helped with the stop motion action sequences, which were very labor-intensive and time-consuming, the voice-over and sound effects, and the final editing using two VHS tapes and recorders as well as the camera. The whole project took a few weeks of LEGO Club sessions to complete, but the final product was accepted by the member's teacher, and he was given an A for it, and the other group members were inspired by the whole process. Not only were the group members impressed, but children who were attending other groups went to see the film (as did their parents and siblings), and virtually everyone who saw it began sharing their own short, animated LEGO film ideas.

Once the option of participating in a LEGO stop-motion animated film became available, many LEGO Club participants chose to focus their efforts on doing that as opposed to elaborate LEGO structural creations. The advent of widespread social media access for this age group facilitated the dissemination of LEGO-based animated films, and making LEGO movies quickly became a popular pastime. This is a good example of the normal process of growth in degrees of freedom that occur in synergistic systems; LEGO animated films represent an unpredicted, emergent outcome of LEGO play activities which themselves now have a wide range of variables and parameters. For LEGO Club participants, this new level or system of LEGO play offers an expanded range and diversity of roles. Rather than having helpers, part-suppliers, pre-assemblers, builders, designers, and engineers, the LEGO

Club activities now involve all those roles plus screenwriters, set-designers, voice actors, cinematographers, stop-motion animators, story-board designers, directors, editors, and special-effects technicians.

The stop-motion animation process using LEGO also led to an expansion of the external system involvement. Many more children at schools and young adults at college are familiar with or may have participated in LEGO stop motion animation. Although most children have been familiar with LEGO materials for many decades now, it was not considered socially normal or acceptable for adults to admit to being LEGO fans. That has changed dramatically in just the past decade now that an entire generation of children has grown up and become adults and parents themselves have watched LEGO animated films, have an active and ongoing interest in higher-level LEGO projects, and participate in their own stop-motion animation projects at home with their families. Stop-motion filming and editing software is now easily accessed using smart-phone technology and many apps can be downloaded for free. The opportunity to share self-made short films on YouTube, Instagram, Tik-Tok and other social media venues is also widely available. There are now social media sites dedicated to sharing amateur LEGO-based stop-motion animated films.

The use of LEGO as a material for creating media productions with sets, scenes, props, and characters all made with LEGO expanded the range of skillful self-expression, but it also increased the level of complexity and challenges for social communication and collaboration. There is a greater diversity of roles, responsibilities, tasks, and feedback loops, with many tasks being dependent on the effective execution of directly or indirectly related other tasks, such as set building being dependent on scripts and storyboards, and voice-over acting relying on sound editing, or stop-motion animation relying on special effects techniques and editing. These are all dynamic operations within the system that are new and emerged because of the creativity of a few group members who first had the idea of using LEGO as a stop-motion material for a school history project.

Just as the specific roles and relationships within the original triad model of set-building has become a tradition within LEGO Club, the objective of developing the LEGO-based and interpersonal skills needed to participate in LEGO stop-motion animation projects has become a tradition. LEGO for many children and most young adult fans is not just about creating three-dimensional structures with bricks; movies are an accepted part of the culture of LEGO today. The specific details of how to offer LEGO stop-motion animation as a project for LEGO Club participants is not a topic in this manual for a reason. The same reason that this manual does not contain instructions on how to build LEGO sets or to do freestyle creations: the point of LEGO Club is not to teach children how to play LEGO, but how to play with each other. That process itself is highly motivating if the activities are of interest to the participants. They will figure out how to build the LEGO sets, create freestyle structures, and make scenes and stop-motion films if they are given the materials and a group of peers. What LBT does is facilitate social interactions and communication by unobtrusively coaching them from the sidelines.

The level system in LEGO Club. The following description of the LEGO Club level system is one that occurred in various groups over time in natural and organic progression as the members and their groups progressed in their skills and proficiency with LEGO and each other. It is not meant to indicate how therapists should structure the group, other than to provide some useful advice about how to communicate about achievements with group members, including the offering of certificates of achievement which offer recognition from the therapist, the other group members, and the group for accomplishing a given level of skill. The LBT model views a child's development as expanding the internal prediction and control over degrees of freedom of the events of systems that are relevant to a child's adaptive functioning. The LBT model also holds that children who benefit from this form of therapy are those for whom interpersonal communication and sociocultural norms are systems for which they have not already internalized adequate familiarity or shared values. This is not the same goal as helping children who have intact abilities to participate in sociocultural systems but for other reasons are disruptive or engage in maladaptive patterns in those settings.

For that reason, the level system in LEGO Club is more predictable and beneficial than would otherwise be expected for children with a broad range of social adjustment issues. Autistic children or children with other internalization problems—children who are withdrawn from or have experienced exclusion from sociocultural systems—benefit from this approach and this structural model of intervention. While children with other types of socialization problems may also benefit from this model, having them participate with autistic children in LEGO Club has not been demonstrated to be beneficial. Based on the understanding of LEGO Club as an opportunity to experience interpersonal identification and shared accomplishment in a synergistic, collaborative sociocultural system, having children with different interpersonal styles and social adjustment issues in the same group is clearly not going to be successful.

As mentioned above, while some children move quickly through the early levels, it is still important for them to demonstrate and receive peer recognition for their achievement of these accomplishments and skillsets. Also keep in mind that each level has a LEGO skillset as well as a social one, and the social goals are more important from a therapeutic point of view than the LEGO-based skills. In a large, busy LEGO Club it can be difficult to keep track of which members have achieved which levels, but from personal experience, it is often much more important and easier for the participants themselves to keep track of what levels they are working on and which certificates they have received. Note that the description of the LEGO-based skills and the interpersonal and communication skills for each level are what members at that level need to demonstrate to other members to be given a certificate for that level and move on to the next.

Designing and printing simple LEGO Club certificates for each level, with space for signatures for each group member and the therapist, is not a complex or problematic process these days. Microsoft Word has some good options for diploma or certificate formats, and there are many others available for free online. The printing and presentation of a LEGO Certificate for a participant who has achieved a given level should include involvement and input from parents, and this is certainly a good opportunity for LEGO Club members to share their accomplishments with their families and other social supports. The main emphasis for the group members should be on the group recognition of the valuable contributions, so before a certificate is awarded, the other group members should agree about the criteria for achieving it and their observations of the group member's participation which had made them eligible to receive it.

Helper. The LEGO Helper level is the entry point for all new LEGO Club members. A group member does not need to earn a Helper certificate. Prior to being introduced to a group they should have had adequate time with the therapist to review the LEGO Club procedures including the LEGO Club Rules, the appropriate Rules of Cool, the common activities (set-building, freestyle creating, and stop-motion filmmaking), and the Level System. They should understand that they will be expected to demonstrate the skill sets of the LEGO Helper and Builder levels, both LEGO-based and interpersonal and communication skills, before they will be allowed to participate in activities and responsibilities at the Creator, Expert, or Genius levels. Their job as helpers is to support the activities in the group and accomplish the tasks assigned to them by the therapist or other group members, especially the leaders who will be at the Creator, Expert and Genius level, or mentors at the LEGO Legend level. By doing so, they will demonstrate their skills that will allow them to become an effective LEGO Builder.

- *LEGO Skills*—Sorting and organizing freestyle bricks. Searching for bricks by color, shape, size, or function. Putting bricks back in the correct bins after use, disassembling sets, or freestyle creations into loose bricks. Pre-assembly or simple building tasks. Participating in stop-motion filming in prescribed ways as stop-motion animator, voice actor, or special effects generator (e.g., making noises, or vocalizing on cue, throwing things into scenes, or shaking a table), or assisting with lighting, or other simple equipment use. Following set directions on simple sets (up to 100 bricks) with minimal support. Selecting correct bricks based on directions. Placement of bricks in correct position based on set directions. Checking LEGO sets for integrity (missing or incorrect pieces) based on the set directions. Helping with clean up.
- *Interpersonal & Communication Skills*—Following the LEGO Club proscriptive rules and understanding the Rules of Cool (not demonstrating them, just understanding that they are there). Communicate with others appropriately and identify the group leaders. Listening attentively to directions and following them. Following directions and staying on task. Being on time for the group and leaving on time without being disruptive in the group or waiting room settings. Not being disruptive and not introducing non-LEGO elements, including actions which are not part of LEGO Club activities, into the room. Communication skills are mostly receptive, but basic forms of verbal and/or gestural communication are necessary to move up to LEGO Builder.

Builder. Once a group member earns a LEGO Builder certificate, they also earn the opportunity to demonstrate their knowledge of the LEGO system and building skills so that they can move up to the next level, LEGO Creator. As a builder, they take responsibility for accurate building of sets, including the basic triad of building skills. The important challenges for a Builder to move up to taking on the challenges of being a Creator include better interpersonal skills including an emphasis on effective nonverbal communication and collaboration. While Helpers often require a lot of direction and input other group members about how to complete basic building tasks, LEGO Builders should be able to take on these tasks collaboratively and without redirection or corrective feedback before they move on to the LEGO Creator level.

- *LEGO Skills*—Assist with opening the boxes and bags for new sets and putting the LEGO bricks from a set onto trays. Sorting the LEGO parts of sets according to form and function and preparing or pre-assembling bricks. Initiating the building process for a set by finding the starting point in the directions. Refraining from overstepping their assigned role in a set-building activity, i.e., when assigned as a builder, part-supplier, or engineer on a set-building project, they stay in that role, until directed to switch roles. Able to competently participate in building small to moderate-sized LEGO sets (>100 bricks). Also participates in following directions from higher-level group members on construction of freestyle creations. Can participate in stop-motion film set creation, stop-motion animator tasks, and other tasks like the LEGO Helpers, but can also be responsible for set-building or following a set-designer's instructions. Builders are also adept at recognizing what is or is not a LEGO brick or set piece, and can sort out non-LEGO, as well as clean LEGO bricks, and sort through donated LEGO materials without supervision.
- *Interpersonal & Communication Skills*—LEGO Builders show increased levels of eye contact, facial expression, and gestures in functional ways, and show respect for other group members' roles, interpersonal space, and rarely if ever violate the LEGO Club Rules. LEGO Builders should have some awareness of the Rules of Cool, such as being able to list at least a couple of them or identify when a Rule of Cool might be needed or when one was being violated by themselves or another group member. Builders should be attending group sessions consistently and learning other group member's names, interests, and proficiency levels before moving on to LEGO Creator.

Creator. At this level, the emphasis for the new LEGO Creator shifts from mostly LEGO building skills to explicitly include interpersonal and communication skills. The challenge for this level has shifted over time from how it was described in the first LBT manual (LeGoff, *et al*, 2014). That description emphasized the creative LEGO skills, building a freestyle, rather than the collaboration and communication with peers on that project. That emphasis over time led to LEGO Builders spending time on their own coming up with LEGO creation ideas, designing, and constructing them, often in isolation in the room, or even doing the project at home and bringing it in to show the group members, both of which technically met the criteria for the LEGO Creator level certificate. In the past ten years, it has become important for all LEGO Club activities to involve joint activity and collaboration, so the LEGO Creator should be required to share a creative idea with the therapist and other group members, and then elicit some level of participation from them in assisting them with refining the design, selecting the parts, and then assembling them with some degree of fidelity to the original idea and design.

- *LEGO Skills*—The LEGO Creator needs to be able to use what they have internalized about the degrees of freedom of the LEGO system in innovative and creative ways. They need to demonstrate an understanding of the redundant degrees of freedom of LEGO bricks; they can be used in multiple ways, and that there is more than one way to achieve a given effect or outcome using different LEGO materials. LEGO Creators maintain their skill and knowledge base for LEGO Builder tasks but add to those the ability to modify LEGO sets or create innovative, novel creations which reflect some of the same design principles. They recognize what is or is not an effective use of LEGO bricks. Come up with novel forms or innovative applications of LEGO. Create a LEGO structure or meet the functional demands of other group members who may be interested in adding elements to a larger freestyle build, or add a structure, vehicle, or piece of equipment to a LEGO scene. Design and engineer LEGO freestyle creations that have face validity—other members recognize its form and function without explanation.
- *Interpersonal & Communication Skills*—Understands, accepts, and follows the LEGO Club rules consistently. Can introduce new group members to the rules. Attends consistently and is not disruptive. Participates in LEGO Club group activities without being disruptive or breaking off from the group to do their own projects. Refrains from proposing inefficient or excessively time- or material-dependent builds which are not realistic for

that group. Accepts feedback from other group members about both their participation in LEGO activities and interpersonal communication and interaction. Uses language to communicate, when necessary, but in general can communicate ideas and needs effectively without adult support and without being disruptive to the group. Can exchange favors with group members and can elicit support for their creative ideas by communicating them effectively, and supporting their ideas with evidence that they are worthwhile and plausible.

Expert. Like the other levels, when a LEGO Creator is given the status of LEGO Expert, they are expected to focus carrying forward the knowledge and skills of the Helper and Builder levels, while consolidating their skills as a Creator by taking on more of a leadership role. This increases the component of increased social and communication skills at a much higher level, allowing them to assume a leadership or executive role in the group. Those group members who have achieved LEGO Creator and are working on LEGO Expert skills show an awareness of how the LEGO Club operates, and not just on projects. They understand how the LEGO materials are acquired and have a sense of the budget and acquisition process involved, and they demonstrate awareness that LEGO Club is a beneficial process with emergent outcomes, not just a place to play with LEGO with some other children.

The extent to which LEGO Club group members have insight into their own goals for participation and how they and others benefit from it is somewhat dependent on the age and developmental level of the members. It is important to keep in mind that the determination of progress from one level to the next should involve a strong emphasis on peer input, so that decision will inevitably involve moderated by age and developmental level since the peers should be similar in these respects. This is especially important for the decision about whether a group member has attained the Expert level because this level emphasizes prosocial and positive interactions with peers, even while taking a leadership role.

- *LEGO Skills*—Incorporating what they have learned about the LEGO system from being a Helper and Builder, the LEGO Expert looks for opportunities to take the lead on modifying or improving designs, helping other group members with design and engineering problems, and generating new project ideas. One of the main tasks of LEGO Experts is problem solving on projects and deciding how best to use available materials to achieve the form and function demands of group projects. They also look for opportunities to offer designs which the group can work on which they can take a leadership role and thereby convince the group members that they are able to move up to the LEGO Genius level.

- *Interpersonal & Communication Skills*—At this level, the group members should have a realistic sense of what is achievable within a certain time (a LEGO session or series of LEGO sessions) to help guide the planning of activities. LEGO Creators who are ready to become LEGO Experts have demonstrated that they recognize the abilities and skills of the other group members, and they collaborate by eliciting input and contributions from them. LEGO Creators reach the Expert level by encouraging participation in diverse ways, not taking over a task, trying to outshine or dominate an activity, and assigning complementary tasks to others. LEGO Experts need to be good delegators of responsibility, as well as taking on higher-level responsibility for operational tasks such as time management, problem-solving, and conflict resolution among group members. The LEGO Expert, who is ready to become a LEGO Genius not only accepts the LEGO Rules, and knows about the Rules of Cool, but actively assists other group members to follow them.

Genius. The LEGO Genius level and the next level, LEGO Legend, evolved from earlier LBT level systems which ended at the LEGO Expert level. The impetus for the LEGO Genius level came from some group participants who had achieved the LEGO Expert level but either wanted to continue to attend so that they could continue to work on projects, or they recognized that they still needed to improve their interpersonal and communication skills. By the time a group member had achieved LEGO Expert level, there were no LEGO building or design skills which they had not achieved. The decision to add the Genius level also came from parents and other professionals who recognized that there were social challenges in the group members' lives which involved interpersonal themes and conflicts (degrees of freedom) which were beyond the skillset involved in collaboration and communication with peers.

The interpersonal and sociocultural challenges that were faced by LEGO Club members who had become LEGO Experts were not those of the classroom or workplace, necessarily, but of interpersonal relationships, coherent emotional expressions, and self-regulation, sharing of life experiences, following social norms in relationships of different types, and the capacity for deeper interpersonal connection. At the LEGO Expert level, we found that group members were able to focus on those issues in part through their continued participation in the LEGO Club—not just with other group members, but with their families and their friends—as well as through the expressive medium of the LEGO filmmaking. Group members who move on from being LEGO Experts to being LEGO Geniuses participate in communication with other group members about their personal lives, their social and emotional conflicts. They also can express their awareness of sociocultural issues, using drama, humor, and symbolic representation in a more mature therapeutic way. In this way, activities at the LEGO Expert level leading to the LEGO Genius level are more like traditional forms of expressive therapy and group psychotherapy.

- *LEGO Skills*—LEGO Experts who are attaining a LEGO Genius level need to be adept at identifying the skills and knowledge base of other group members. They retain all their own skills and knowledge of LEGO as a system to help them find ways to improve the level of the group. LEGO Experts create the scaffolding for other group members' achievement of higher abilities and skills by offering insights about the LEGO system, as well as their knowledge and past experiences with LEGO materials. LEGO Experts who become LEGO Geniuses can participate in all levels of LEGO activities and contribute to those activities without needing to show that they are better than others; they demonstrate humility and generosity, while also taking leadership, solving problems, and making decisions when necessary.
- *Interpersonal & Communication Skills*—Designating tasks to group members based on those other members' abilities, skills, and knowledge is important at this level. LEGO Experts who are working on attaining LEGO Genius status are typically engaged in helping others with their LEGO projects as advisors, or they are working on their own LEGO stop-motion film projects. In that context, they come up with short film ideas, either new ones, or scripts, songs, or other media, like stand-up comedy routines, music-videos, or LEGO replications of children's story books, fairytales, historical events, etc. LEGO Geniuses take creative ideas from other group members or their own and break them down into achievable projects as

part of an overall project management approach. They allocate responsibilities as needed and take responsibility for each component of a project like the script, storyboard, set-designs, set-building, camera angles and special effects, and sound effects. If necessary, they hold auditions and rehearsals for the voice actors, and do run-throughs of action sequences with the stop-motion animators. The main tasks of the LEGO Genius are to generate group synergy by keeping group members focused and collaborating on a project, keeping a record, and providing a sense of continuity and commitment to the overall project so that other group members do not lose track of their responsibilities and commitment to the project. They also address interpersonal conflicts and any individual issues which may come up with group members which interferes with the group activity or with that group member's participation.

LEGO Legend. Once a group member has achieved the LEGO Genius level, they will have contributed a body of work to the LEGO Club in terms of maintaining the Club's materials, establishing relationships with other group members and their families, large set building projects, freestyle creations, and stop-motion animated films. With modern media, these accomplishments are often evident on the Club's website or other media postings, as well as in the LEGO room itself if there is one. The LEGO Genius and LEGO Legend levels are not commonly attained in groups which have time-limited enrollment, or which occur in institutional settings like residential placements or schools, due to the time constraints. These levels, however, are important and contribute significantly to the overall effectiveness of outpatient clinics or other private settings (e.g., private schools), where LEGO Club participation can be open-ended.

Once a LEGO Genius graduates to the level of LEGO Legend, they are not considered a group member so much as a group mentor. This "level," is really a different role which emerged when some LEGO Club members who achieved both LEGO Expert and then LEGO Genius status still wanted to maintain their affiliation with the group and continue to participate, but they were already at or above age level on their social and communication skills and adaptive socialization goals. The LEGO Legend role is an opportunity for former group members to consolidate their acquired social competence by helping other children. They are invited to participate in their former group, or in any other groups as volunteer mentors and help the therapists by supporting the LEGO-based activities as well as the interpersonal and communication skill development of the members.

In my experience, some LEGO Legends enjoy working with the younger group members on their set-building and freestyle projects, or they may want to maintain a connection with their friends in the more advanced groups, or work on LEGO stop motion films together and stay in touch via social media. The LEGO Legend role demonstrates the real-world value that group members give to the LEGO Club as a social group, and not simply as a form of intervention. Depending on the age and educational level of the group member, LEGO Legends may need to have their parents' permission to continue to participate, but the usual arrangements for therapeutic fees or group membership fees are normally waived. They are volunteer mentors, not participants. In school settings, this would create complications if a LEGO Legend had graduated from the school, of course, but there are peer mentor programs which could be set up to accommodate LEGO Clubs at many high schools and colleges. Some group members have also continued to participate in a form of LEGO Club as a group therapy for young adults, in which the LEGO activities are optional or an expressive medium for more psychotherapeutic goals of the group. This would not be referred to as "LEGO Club," however, since that might be confusing for the group members. Offering support groups or group therapy for autistic young adults is another topic, not part of LBT, but the objectives of those services could be seen as a continuation of the LEGO Club model, consistent with the overall goals of LBT.

CHAPTER 8

FACILITATING SOCIAL DEVELOPMENT DURING LEGO CLUB ACTIVITIES

L EGO-Based Therapy and child development are organic processes. Although LBT involves some degree of adult direction and professional facilitation, the sessions also reflect developmental processes that are organic in the sense of arising from genetic and cultural influences which derive from human evolutionary history, getting together and engaging in culturally relevant, creative play has always been an element of not just child development but human development. Before humans formed social structures that were large and complex enough to allow for the creation of schools, children learned by playing together. Play is like bread; if you put the basic ingredients together to get it going and do not interfere with it, it just happens. This is like all forms of organic growth, and life as a system on our planet; if humans do not interfere with it, it will continue to happen.

Of course, humans are organisms, and the social and cultural systems which we have created to help us survive and flourish all over the planet are based on the same organic principles as life itself. There are elements of sociocultural systems, and whole systems which have emerged from them, which are not based on organic principles and values. For us as humans, life, and experiences of life, are of the highest value. Without life, nothing has value, at least from the point of view of living organisms. That point is easily lost if we become distracted by systems which have other values, the most common of which is economics. Economic systems arise from sociocultural systems and were developed to support them; we invented money and forms of exchange to facilitate trade which is important for the diversity and sustainability of sociocultural systems. Economics, however, has values that do not overlap with life or life experience. Economic systems only influence life through the intermediary effects on sociocultural systems.

That may seem like a very distant and abstract discussion relative to setting up LBT, but in fact, it is relevant. Economic factors are a reality of both setting up and running LBT, and it is a reality of child development. Therapists are as aware and responsible as teachers, parents, and those more directly involved in weighing children's developmental needs against economic factors, school administrators, school boards, and those in charge of developmental and educational agencies. One of the arguments made in the previous book about applied behavior analysis (LeGoff, 2023), is directly relevant to the issue of how economic pressures may be negatively influencing child development, especially as it relates to autistic children. There are now large and highly developed markets for ABA-based services, and other intensive forms of intervention, which provide economic support for profitable private providers who can afford to market their services to large audiences and promote misinformation about autism and the benefit of their services. Quite often they have no credible evidence that what they are selling has any benefit to either our sociocultural systems or to the life experience of the children involved, but they continue to thrive in economic terms.

Without having to get into any sort of detailed economic analysis, it is obvious that LBT has a low cost-to-benefit ratio compared with other forms of intervention. This is especially true if we focus on addressing the important underlying issues for autistic children and their families, or other developmentally and socially diverse groups who may need additional support for learning how to participate effectively in sociocultural systems. In that regard, "participating in sociocultural systems," involves learning how to communicate, interact, and use the technological advantages that are available to all citizens of a given society. As was written earlier, LEGO Club provides a play-based microcosm of these sociocultural systems and their synergistic dynamics. The main problem with many other forms of intervention targeted at the autism services market—aside from the obvious economic costs and negative impact on life experiences of those involved—is that they are not themselves based on an organic model of sociocultural development.

To some extent, how we interact with and educate autistic children must consider what we know about typical child development. It is not enough to say that neurodiverse or socially diverse children are not typical and therefore intervention strategies must be based on strategies other than the normal processes involved in children's sociocultural development. What that approach misunderstands is that education has never replaced play and social learning in typical children but exists alongside it as an institutional form of learning. Educational curricula allow for social development, they do not interfere with it, but they are not the cause of it. There is no cause for children's sociocultural development unless we consider *being a child* a cause. Thinking about child development using cause-effect models also misses the point that children are as much the causes of sociocultural systems as the reverse. Social groups and culture are emergent outcomes of interpersonal relationships, both ontogenetically— for the developing child—and phylogenetically—for our developing species (Grandqvist, 2021; Muthukrishna, *et al*, 2018; Creanza, *et al*, 2017; Burghardt, 2015; Foley & Lahr, 2011; LaFreniere, 2011; van Schaik & Burkhart, 2011; Pinker, 2010; Smith & Kirby, 2008; Whiten & van Schaik, 2007; Gaskins, *et al*, 2006; Goncu & Gaskins, 2006; Smith, 2006; Geary, 2005; Hamilton, 1964). Having fun by playing together is not something children do when school is over, it is at the core of what has allowed our species to survive and what will be responsible for our organic, social, and cultural future.

For most children, the process of learning and development through participating in play with peers happens naturally without any professional oversight or facilitation. This is likely to become a normal process for children who do not develop in typical ways over time; in other words, culture and education will eventually adapt and accommodate neurodiversity. In the meantime, though, there appear to be elements within those systems (possibly maintained by external economic factors) that can be described as antergistic; they maintain or exacerbate a maladaptive outcome. That is the current situation with the identification and excessive intervention associated with the diagnosis and treatment of autism spectrum disorder (ASD). Rather than viewing developmentally diverse children as needing some accommodations or supports (adaptations) for them to participate in their sociocultural systems—benefitting from and contributing to those systems—the medical and behavioral models of ASDs construe neurodiversity using a disease model (within medical science), or as a form of maladaptive learned behavior (in the ABA model).

Ironically, the justification for using the medical and behavioral model of ASD in technologically advanced democratic societies is that not doing so would result in developmental and educational discrimination. The goal of special education laws in the US (*the Individuals with Disabilities Education Act*, IDEA, 2004), has been to promote equal access to and meaningful benefit from societal sources of developmental and educational benefits. These laws have been used to justify the identification of children with disabilities, and implementation of what the system has determined are beneficial interventions based on research on what are known as best practices. Unfortunately, there have been multiple maladaptive factors involved in the determination and implementation of best practices including short-sighted definitions of educational benefits (i.e., behavioral goals), and biased opinions about efficacy of services due to overly narrow and self-interested research (i.e., ABA-based, and pharmacological studies). As a result of these maladaptive influences, the focus of administrative efforts has been to improve the availability of ABA services and psychotropic medications, not the cost-benefit assessment of those interventions for children, families, and society at large.

This message is directed more towards administrators and those who influence the allocation of funding for services in family services, healthcare, and education, but it is also important for therapists, educators, and parents to know what they may be up against, and how they can promote LBT as a cost-effective, less invasive alternative to ABA or pharmacological interventions. The anticipated rebuttal argument to promoting LBT is that it will not be as immediately effective as either ABA services or psychotropic medications. That is a superficial and almost meaningless argument since "effective," is defined by the professionals who are promoting and financially benefitting from those services. School administrators and others may be supportive of the short-term benefit they define as decreased rates of non-compliant behavior in the classroom, to which the example of LEGO Club can be offered: the children want to be there and are willing to abide by the rules to participate. The counterargument to that is that we cannot make all classrooms into LEGO Clubs, which is another invalid argument because, obviously, we can. There is no reason that classrooms cannot be designed to facilitate the socio-cultural synergistic dynamics of LEGO Club using the principles of LBT. These are not significantly different from the principles of constructivism, which are widely used in all educational settings (Gunduz & Hersen, 2015; Wadsworth, 2004).

Some behavior analytic writers claim that "naturalistic" ABA methods are compatible with constructivist models of learning and development (Schreibman, *et al*, 2015). Hybrid models of constructivism and ABA seem to be a worthwhile idea on the surface, but in fact, with a deeper look at the level of basic values and conceptualization of learning and development, these are diametrically opposed views and are not compatible at all. Constructivism construes learning and development as the emergent outcome of the internal systems of individuals benefiting from and contributing to their external sociocultural environments. It is an organic model of growth, not a linear cause-effect model, with the cause of learning being external events and the effect being changes in behavior. Even the definition of the objectives is incompatible. Behaviorism and ABA exclude cognitive processes from their causal model, while constructivists identify cognitive processes as central to learning and development.

Behavior analysts focus their interventions on the environment—reinforcement schedules of behaviors—while constructivists focus on the system as a whole: children's initiation of understanding and acting upon their social and physical environment, and that environment's facilitation of learning through providing the opportunity for playful learning and creativity. Vygotsky was right to identify the developmental process as a sociohistorical one which includes human evolutionary history. Play and learning are part of our genetic and cultural evolutionary history, not an individual child's environmental reinforcement history. This stark contrast between models is even more apparent when we consider the cost-benefit analysis of using psychoactive medications to alter the neurochemical functioning of a child's brain. That is a decision that should be left up to a child's parents and their pediatrician or child psychiatrist, but it is remarkable how many parents find themselves consulting physicians about psychopharmacological options for their child because their educational staff suggested it. There may be reasons for parents and physicians to consider using psychoactive medications to help a child to focus, learn, or to gain more self-control in stimulating situations, but as has been argued elsewhere (LeGoff, 2023), being autistic is not a behavior problem. Viewing neurodiverse children through the lens of ABA or psychopharmacology, however, might lead one to believe that misconception.

Facilitating the organic process. Children, like all organisms, are genetically designed to operate within certain ecosystems or niches which themselves are systems with identifiable degrees of freedom, parameters, and dynamic, homeostatic operations. Humans are physiologically and neurologically complex organisms and they do not develop, and function based on their genetic makeup alone; in fact, most of the important adaptive strategies we use only start with genetics and are supplanted by learning through experience and social learning—imitation, modeling, verbal, and nonverbal symbolic communication—in early childhood. In fact, humans need to learn to survive beyond infancy. As parents, educators, and therapists we do not need to know precisely how children learn through experiences of their environments to facilitate their development, but we still need to facilitate their development. That was the point that Donald Winnicott emphasized when he famously said, "There is no such thing as an infant." Without a facilitating environment, infants do not survive.

It is also true to say that without a facilitating environment, most infants and children do not learn and develop. That is not entirely true, however, with respect to autistic children. What many people, including many developmental, educational, and healthcare professionals, view as "symptoms of autism," may be more correctly viewed as evidence of children learning and developing without the influence of sociality. Recall that sociality is a normally distributed trait of anthropocentrism which is expressed as a bias in attention and learning towards sociocultural events. In other words, typical humans' infants are born being predisposed to value other people and events in the environment around them involving other people—their actions and actions with objects—more than events that do not involve people or cultural objects. Autistic and other developmentally diverse children may not have this bias, and as a result, they tend to focus on all events—physical or anthropological—resulting in less of a bias towards sociocultural events. They are less anthropocentric to begin with, and that leads to them following developmentally divergent pathways.

This early difference in sociality is complicated by another related factor which is also not a characteristic of being autistic or developmentally diverse but is characteristic which specific to typically developing infants and children. That is the decrease in alerting response which results from adult, especially parental, social contact. There is considerable research to show that in typical children, the subcortical brain structure which regulates their innate attending to environmental events, the alerting or orienting response, is selectively inhibited by the presence of their parents. That means that most children will ignore whatever else might be going on around them when their parents are nearby, and it allows them to stay calm and focused on them—their facial expressions, hand actions and actions-with-objects, their voices, etc., and not everything else (Andrews, *et al*, 2022; Simic, *et al*, 2021; Bernaerts, *et al*, 2020; Bannerjee, *et al*, 2016; Chau & Galvez, 2012; Ashwin, *et al*, 2007; Sander, Grafman & Zalla, 2003; Adolphs & Tranel, 2000; Baron Cohen, *et al*, 2000). It has also been established that chronic over-activation and growth of the amygdala is associated with autistic development (Herrington, *et al*, 2017; Zala & Sperduti, 2013; Schumann, *et al*, 2011; 2009; 2004).

Citing the research literature on infant attachment and amygdala functioning in autistic children may seem like an abstract and indirect way to describe how one should facilitate social development in a LEGO Club, there are some pragmatic and direct implications of this research for LBT. What we understand based on the neuroscience of infant orienting responses (amygdala activation), and learning is that all children can learn how to participate in sociocultural systems if they are in a calm, safe environment where they can play, and their attention is drawn to events (actions and objects) as sociocultural events. That means their attention is focused on the people and cultural objects so that they can learn how they can participate in those relationships. Playful learning requires that children feel calm and safe, so that they are not goal-directed or defended, which is the result of being in unfamiliar and unpredictable environments. Not feeling safe, welcome, and engaged by an environment—both social and physical—inhibits the natural processes of self-initiated play and learning.

The anxiety and stress which inhibit play and learning in children arises from unpredictable environmental events which often carry negative consequences. The therapeutic benefit of being a member of LEGO Club is partly due to its disconfirming experiences. The anticipation of unpredictable negative events is disconfirmed as a pessimistic expectation first by the presentation of an inherently fun activity with which the child can identify some sense of belonging and meaning. Second, the therapist and other group members introduce new group members to the rules and routines of the group, with no hidden agendas or unforeseen consequences. Children in LEGO Club do not have to "work to earn rewards," as they do in settings controlled by behavior analysts. Participating in LEGO Club is simply fun and there is no cost to the child for participating, other than contributing to their interest, efforts, and creativity. Finally, the expectations of the peers and interactions with them are not mysterious, emotional, or fraught with conflict. The therapist and the other children outline the agenda in advance and give gentle reminders about social norms and communication in ways that are helpful and not humiliating or frustrating.

The work that the therapist does is often in advance of the group sessions, not during them. In other discussions of the LBT, the therapists' role during the group session has been described as that of a border collie herding sheep. That is not to compare the children's activity to that of sheep in a herd, but to highlight the therapist's actions as maintaining a boundary for the LEGO Club system. The therapists are neither group members, nor are they external to the group. The therapists determine what goes into the LEGO Club—the children and materials—not what happens in the LEGO Club—the activities and interactions.

The therapist maintains a neutral stance with respect to interpersonal conflicts of the group members, and like any other form of expressive or play therapy, does not press, or interfere with the process even when insights, growth, and change seem to be painfully slow to come. The most important task of the therapist in LBT, aside from selecting the group members and setting up the session and materials, is unobtrusively encouraging the group members to communicate and collaborate with each other, and especially to give feedback about social and emotional issues. The members will be able to work out what to do with the LEGO themselves; what they need some hints and prompting about will be what to do with each other.

As was described previously (LeGoff, 2023, 2017; LeGoff, et al, 2014; 2011; 2010), it is helpful to introduce a child to the LEGO Club model individually at first, establishing a trusting and supportive relationship with the therapist before introducing them to a group. Consequently, it is not surprising that new group members will frequently turn to the therapist for input and support when they start attending. It is important to maintain that alliance, but to also build upon it by first introducing the new group member to the others, and then encouraging them to approach the others when they need help or have questions. That, of course, could go badly if the other group members were not previously prepared and willing to be helpful to the new group member, or if the group is just starting and all the members are new.

That is why it is preferable not to start a LEGO Club with all new group members joining at the same time. In my experience, that problem is easily overcome by starting a group with just a couple of group members. The first two members should be children who have at least the potential to become the group's first leaders, who can communicate with other members about the rules, expectations, and activities, and they should also be highly motivated and familiar enough with LEGO to expect that they will sustain their group membership over time. The next step would be to start adding individual group members one at a time, with at least a LEGO Club or two for the new members to begin to feel like they belong and are part of the Club before adding another member. While starting a group with five or six members right away is possible, and has been done many times, the social dynamics are difficult to keep track of, and there are inevitably more initial conflicts and negative interactions resulting in a lingering sense of mistrust or dread going forward that negative events are inevitable, and that negative expectation can take a long time to overcome.

Structuring LEGO Club Sessions. The format of LEGO sessions has been described elsewhere (LeGoff, 2017; LeGoff, *et al*, 2014), but this aspect of the successful implementation of LBT is so critical it bears repeating. The LBT therapist is encouraged to anticipate all aspects of the group members' experience, not just the session itself. The timing of the group session may create conflicts for individual members, so it is worthwhile discussing with the member and their parents the group schedule and what else may be going on for them at that time. If parents must get off early from work and travel to the child's school to get them, and then have a long trip to the clinic, there are inevitably going to be problems sustaining that arrangement, and it could result in an unacceptable level of cost in terms of stress for both the parent and the child. This is also true for students who may attend LEGO Club groups at their school. Some attention needs to be paid to having the child attend LEGO Club groups when it is not going to interfere with other important or valued activities.

If a therapist is hosting more than one session on a given day, be sure to allow adequate time in between sessions to allow for group members and their families to leave, and for the therapy room to be readied for the next group. The LEGO Club materials should be available and ready for use when group members arrive. They should be encouraged to spend the initial few minutes of every session discussing Club business—new group members may need to be introduced, the group members' levels should be reviewed and discussed, if a group member is getting ready to graduate to the next level, or if someone is leaving the group this needs to be discussed, upcoming events (birthdays, graduations, holidays), new LEGO acquisitions and budgeting should be reviewed, and the social media coverage of group activities should be updated. Finally, the group should discuss and agree on the chosen activity and objectives for that session.

The LEGO Club activity should remain the bulk of the activity and main objective of the group session, but it is also sometimes therapeutic to allow group members to engage in interaction and discussion about relevant Club issues, even if that ends up taking most of the Club's session time. If the group members would prefer to spend their time socializing, joking around, or arguing with each other, that is normal and should not be interfered with by the therapist prompting them to get on with a LEGO project. The LEGO activities are engaged in to facilitate social communication, not the other way around. The parents, family members, and other interested parties should also be prepared for the possibility that the LEGO Club did not build any LEGO sets but spent the group time arguing about the plot in a planned LEGO film, discussing one the group member's problems at school, or deciding what to do about a new group member's annoying habit.

For the most part, group members will want to get on with the LEGO activities, but they often have short memories for what had been agreed upon in the last session about this session's activity and who would be filling which roles. Each LEGO Club session should end with some time to clean and organize the room, as well as to discuss any problems encountered that day interpersonally and resolve those issues, and then discuss the next week's activity. The therapist or a senior group member should take notes. LEGO Clubs often generate a lot of notes and drawings: scripts, story boards, ideas for projects, drawings of proposed freestyles, spontaneous new proscriptive rules or "Rules of Cool," notes to other groups ("Clean up your messes!" "Stop bringing food into LEGO Club," or "Do not touch!"). These are sometimes just left here and there around the room, put into folders, and filed in a file box, posted on a cork board, or written on a white board, or posted on a LEGO Club website. These communications need to be facilitated and respected by the adults involved as they are important to the continuity and identity of the group, as well as for the social identity of the group members.

CHAPTER 9

FACILITATING SOCIAL DEVELOPMENT OUTSIDE OF THE LEGO CLUB

Families. Participating in LEGO Club is often not the first peer group experience that families of autistic or developmentally diverse children have, but it is often the first successful one. Past negative experiences of social groups typically include negative events in preschool or daycare, church groups, play groups, classrooms, and team sports. The neutral or positive peer-group experiences usually include small special needs settings, Scouts or Guides, martial arts, and swimming. Some children and adolescents have also reported positive experiences with other individual sports like track and field, or activities like hiking/orienteering, climbing, fishing, and paddling. Outdoor activities like these tend to be both healthy and involve natural environments with less emphasis on sociocultural systems (social norms, rules and expectations that are often implied, and involve a high reliance on social imitation and modeling). Aside from LEGO Club, these sorts of activities can be beneficial, but for many families, finding a social activity that does not result in social withdrawal, exclusion, or sheer disaster, is difficult. This is especially true of families who have more than one child.

There is considerable discussion in the autism literature on the benefits and risks of autistic children's siblings. Much of the attention recently has been focused on genetic research, and predicting autistic traits in siblings (Szatmari, *et al*, 2016; Georgiades, *et al*, 2013; Elder, *et al*, 2008), and on autistic traits or the *Broader Autism Phenotype* (BAP, Kellerman, *et al*, 2019; Tsai, *et al*, 2017). There is also some consideration of the impact on siblings of having an autistic brother or sister (Orsmond and Seltzer, 2009), or on the possible benefit that siblings may offer to autistic children (Huskens, *et al*, 2015). Whether siblings of autistic children are themselves autistic, or have some autistic traits, does not necessarily determine whether they can be viewed as a potential resource for the family or not. To some extent this depends on the parents. Some parents are absolutely mystified by having more than one autistic child, and other parents seem to have expected it—to no one's surprise. The rates of autistic traits in parents are another hot topic for genetics research, of course, and for research on offering parenting support and interventions (Crowell, *et al*, 2019).

Genetic studies have a long tradition in autism research (c.f., Thapar & Rutter, 2021; Rutter, 2000). There is also a long tradition of theories about autistic development which identify parenting styles as the cause of the condition, whether it was withholding of emotional support (Bettelheim, 1967) or inadvertent reinforcement of autistic behaviors (Ferster, 1961). From a systems point of view, any theory that identifies a single causal factor to account for something as complex as atypical patterns of social development in children are doomed to fail. That is not to say that identifying the factors, both genetic and experiential, which contribute to the variability in sociality and social adaptation is not worthwhile, since there are potentially useful strategies which can be combined to reverse the antergistic influences of multiple maladaptive influences with the synergistic effects of multiple adaptive influences. While most researchers and clinicians would agree that sociality, the BAP, and being autistic all have some genetic contributing factors, the range of adaptive or maladaptive outcomes for individuals with those genetic risk factors can still vary widely based on both early and later life experiences.

There is no doubt that providing some guidance and support to parents to help their child navigate the complex sociocultural systems involved in child development and education these days is a good idea (Chamberlain, 2017). There is a growing literature on that topic (Chamak & Bonniau, 2016), however, most research over the past few decades has focused on getting parents to use ABA techniques at home to change "autistic behaviors," as opposed to helping them to understand and facilitate their child's social and communication development (Harris & Weiss, 1998; Lovaas, 1993; 1987; 1981). Although Peckett, MacCallum and Knibbs (2016) identified some benefits to mothers of having their parents participate in LEGO Club groups, the group itself is clearly not a form of family intervention. As was previously noted in the original outcome studies on LBT (LeGoff & Sherman, 2006; LeGoff, 2004) described that family therapy sessions were conducted along with individual therapy in addition to the LBT group therapy. It seems to be a consensus among both researchers and clinicians that some form of professional input and support for parents and other family members is beneficial for autistic children and their families, even though this does not imply that families or parents are the cause of autism, the BAP, or low sociality.

Whether therapists who host LEGO Club groups are also involved in consulting with the families who attend, it is an important consideration, especially for families who have a high BAP profile, such as families who have more than one child identified as autistic, or who have either parents or other adult family members identified as having the BAP or autism. The research by Green and his colleagues in the UK, and that of Whitehouse and his colleagues in Australia, cited earlier, are excellent examples of cost-effective and efficient strategies to improve social development in autistic or at-risk children. It seems reasonable to expect that the growing body of clinical research literature on these pre-emptive family-oriented early intervention strategies will continue to grow. Combining parental support and advocacy early on, with appropriate educational supports (as opposed to the antergistic ABA-based discrete trial methods) for social development, and opportunities for continued social development such as LEGO Club, may generate the emergent outcomes of a synergistic adaptive system.

In the meantime, offering families some family counseling, psycho-educational input, and support is a helpful plan along with LEGO Club groups. One of the unexpected side-benefits of the LBT sessions has been the impromptu support networks which have developed among the families whose children attend LBT. Whether it is in the waiting area, or through school or other institutional parent support networks, parents of LEGO Club members tend to respond in ways that are like their children's responses to each other. They identify with each other and have often had similar experiences, but they each have unique histories as well, and sharing those tends to strengthen the sense of belonging, improve their resilience and adaptability, and increase their commitment to the LEGO Club and to each other. This has been especially notable in groups which have taken place over longer periods of time, and in which the families have become familiar with each other and have participated in both positive and negative life events together (LeGoff, 2017). The informal support network and sharing of resources among the parents of LEGO Club participants is also an organic sociocultural outcome and does not need much monitoring or support from the LEGO Club host. In fact, just like LEGO Club sessions, it seems to be that less professional involvement in that process is better.

Schools. LEGO Club groups have been set up and run successfully in school settings in a range of formats, both as an activity within existing classrooms, and on a pull-out basis (Evans & Bond, 2021; Hu, *et al*, 2018; Boyne, 2014; LeGoff, *et al*, 2010). Although I have not conducted any specific studies on school-based LEGO Clubs, I have been involved in setting up and running groups at both private and public schools for many years. This approach does have some advantages over the clinic-based groups, especially for the family, who do not need to get involved in the potentially stressful transportation of children to the clinic as well as not interfering with other family activities. The scheduling is also advantageous to some therapists who may not have much time during the evening or weekend hours to run LEGO Club groups, which are the only times when children can attend without being taken out of school.

Some LEGO Club groups have been set up and run by remedial services providers working in the school system, such as was documented by speech pathologists in the US (Ralph & Rochester, 2016) and occupational therapists in Finland (Hulju & Maki, 2017). Many school districts may not have a budget for LEGO materials, or the space available for a LEGO room, but as mentioned above, economic factors should be discussed openly with school administrators and decision-makers such as regional school boards. The cost of ABA services for autistic preschoolers or primary students, which may be included in their individualized family services plans (IFSPs) or individualized education plans (IEPs), are examples of "evidence-based" interventions whose benefits should be reviewed more carefully. Although LEGO materials are still relatively expensive as a retail product for families, in the context of educational and therapy materials in the budgets of school districts, they are certainly worth considering. LEGO Educational Division also contributes significantly to subsidize the cost of LEGO educational materials for public and private schools internationally. What seems to be more of an issue to expanding the availability of LEGO Club groups in school settings is not the cost of the materials, or even the training, staff hours, or space, but the historical commitment of school-based ABA providers who are resistant to non-ABA interventions.

The initial support for the growth of LBT from one small LEGO Club to an entire program was from educators. Although parents and other family members provided positive feedback about improvements in sociality and social competence among the first LEGO Club members, it was not until I started hearing from educational staff—general education and special education teachers, remedial services providers, and school administrators—about their observations of positive changes in social and play patterns in group members that it seemed likely that LBT was having such a quick and broad-based impact. This feedback was captured in the first LBT publication (LeGoff, 2004), in which the results were derived from classroom, lunchroom and playground observations, as well as teacher and parent ratings. The second, longer-term outcome study (LeGoff & Sherman, 2006) was based on a review of special education assessments that were conducted every three years on children who were participating in LBT. These two studies established right from the outset that the benefits of LBT were not limited to improvements in social interactions and competence with peers in the LEGO Club, but that the participants were showing more general improvements in overall social adaptation.

Although it is often complex and time-consuming to initiate new or different services in a school setting, communicating with schools about the minimal costs and high benefits of LBT is worthwhile. This has been especially fruitful in the past with private schools, and private special education settings, which have more flexibility in their budget and administrative decisions. The clear advantage to those settings is the benefit to the children who participate in effective social development programming, but it is also beneficial for the school since having a LEGO Club can be attractive to potential parents as well as outside funding (e.g., special education and autism services grants). The LEGO Club has also been implemented as an after-school program in both public and private school settings. In one private special needs school, the group was run at the school as an afterschool program but was funded as a group therapy using parents' health insurance.

There are innumerable ways that public and private sectors can collaborate to effectively make LEGO Club groups available through the schools' curriculum, remedial programming, special education services, or afterschool programs. The LEGO Club is also relevant to social development for students across a wide range of needs and ages, from preschool to post-secondary education. Many public and private colleges and universities now offer peer-based support for students with diverse developmental and social needs. The popularity of LEGO activities, including advanced building projects and stop-motion animation, makes them ideal for creating a peer-based support program within student support services, residential services, and as an opportunity for peer mentors in health and social services programs. I have personally been invited to attend LEGO Club groups which have been initiated by professionals but are being run effectively by adolescents and young adults in mainstream high school and college settings.

Communities. In addition to the involvement of a full range of educational settings, LEGO Clubs can be made accessible in community settings, and have been for some time now in public libraries. The history of LEGO Clubs in libraries is quite extensive but seems to have been a grassroots movement among public librarians finding ways to increase the use of their facilities. While this is not associated with implementation of LBT, public libraries being open to hosting LEGO-based group activities is an excellent opportunity to extend the benefits of school or clinic based LBT into a community setting. Aside from the public library LEGO Clubs there are also numerous forms of private organizations which host group LEGO activities for children and adults. While these are usually after-school, weekend, or summer camp programs—designed to give working parents the option of a non-athletic, adult-supervision program—they are also an excellent opportunity for social development. A lot of these groups advertise the cognitive benefits of LEGO play, especially for activities involving more advanced projects and the LEGO robotics materials. That seems to be more related to marketing these programs than any significant benefit in terms of cognitive development or learning capacity.

There are also numerous online resources for both children and adult fans of LEGO. Again, although these are not part of the LBT process, they can add to and support child, adolescent, and young adult participation in sociocultural systems by providing an extension of LBT into publicly available social support networks. Many participants and graduates from LBT over the years have gone on to participate in other LEGO Clubs, both in person and online. The increase in media attention on both individual and group-based LEGO activities has greatly increased the public interest in social and developmental diversity, as well as making the once stigmatizing "idiosyncratic interest," of young adult LEGO fans into a normal social outlet like belonging to any other activity-focused groups like cooking clubs, book clubs, or chess clubs.

There are also many ways for children to participate in community activities through their local church, synagogue, or mosque. Like the public libraries and after-school programs, religious centers have offered to host LEGO-based activities. The obvious benefits for religious organizations include attracting young people to participate in their activities, as well as offering an important stabilizing influence in the community. Therapists, educators, and parents should be aware of these opportunities to extend a child's participation from professionally run LBT groups to more typical sociocultural systems which have a long history of being integrated in the community.

The child and youth scouting organizations, World Organization of the Scout Movement (WOSM), and the World Association of Girl Guides and Girl Scouts (WAGGGS) are represented in most developed countries and are a community-based resource which provides structured goal-directed and peer-mediated learning opportunities. In addition to martial arts, individual sports, and non-therapeutic LEGO Clubs, many of the participants in LBT have transitioned over to the scouting movement successfully. The scouting movement has also begun integrating LEGO into their routines and activities, again with the added benefit for the scout organization of attracting new members and sustaining their motivation for participation.

In general, when the first LBT sessions were held at my office in the mid-1990's, there were not many community-based opportunities for children to participate in LEGO activities with peers. It would also not have been obvious to parents or the adult administrators of LEGO-based groups that LEGO building could be a collaborative activity, and not just an opportunity for parallel play. The rapid expansion of LEGO group-based activities in communities and on the internet may be to some extent a result of LEGO Corporation's marketing and support for group-based activities. LEGO Corporation's administration clearly understands the value of their product being used in this way (I have had that conversation with them in person).

The LEGO Learning Through Play foundation, is a not-for-profit, non-governmental organization supported by LEGO Corporation, now formally involved in supporting both community-based LEGO activities and LBT itself via their sponsorship of Dr. Gina Gomez de la Cuesta's organization, *Play Included*, which offers LBT as the Brick-by-Brick program internationally. The overall goal of the Learning Through Play foundation is to support the United Nation's Sustainable Development Goal 4 (UNSD-4): "Ensure inclusive and equitable access to quality education and promote life-long learning opportunities for all." From the perspective of LBT, the most important part of lifelong learning involves participating in sociocultural systems, which is something that most children and their families can take for granted: they are born with intact sociality and there is no alternative. For autistic children and their families, LBT's small contribution to UNSD-4 may be to "ensure inclusive and equitable access to the social and cultural systems of education and lifelong learning."

CHAPTER 10

BEYOND THE BASICS: ADVANCED TOPICS IN LEGO-BASED THERAPY

Early Learners in LBT. One of the most frequently asked questions I get during LBT workshops and online from those interested in starting LBT groups is about the minimal age of participants. Normally I mention that developmental level is more relevant to age, but the question is the same: at what age-equivalent developmental level can children benefit from participating in LBT? LEGO Corporation takes their product development seriously, and by that I do not mean simply having input from focus groups or using play groups to try out their latest innovations. LEGO's *Learning Through Play* foundation has engaged in highly advanced research on classroom applications, child development, learning, and play involving children from infancy to young adulthood in a wide range of settings internationally (Liu, *et al*, 2017; Whitebread, *et al*, 2017). Their consumer research has included designating the typical age-ranges for which their products are designed, as well as expanding those ranges to include learning and play activities appropriate for younger and older children, as well as to be more inclusive (gender, ethnic, and ability-based diversity has been a recent area of growth).

The good news from the point of view of LBT is that LEGO materials can be utilized by preschoolers, and there is a continuity of that system of play up to adult-level activities. Readers interested in reaching younger children who may have been identified with autistic conditions or who are at risk for autism or the BAP, are encouraged to consider parent-mediated LEGO play as opposed to LBT formally. The limitation for LBT is not the materials themselves, but the fact that typical early learners (infants, up to two years of age) are not yet focused on peers for sociocultural development and are still more focused on adult caregivers. This does not mean that parents should not be encouraged to consider using LEGO to facilitate collaborative play with infants and young children, in fact, using LEGO in this way, as a parent-infant interactive play material is a good option. That approach, however, would not be considered part of LBT, although it has been suggested to Andrew Whitehouse and his colleagues (personal communication).

For the purposes of providing LBT for younger children, a reasonable rule of thumb would be that if children are able to participate in interactive play with peers or siblings, they can participate in LBT. Again, the child's readiness for peer-mediated learning is the limiting factor, not their capacity to engage with LEGO materials. Early forms of interactive play with peers can be combined with increased levels of adult support and direction, as well as modifying the LEGO-based activities to emphasize simple peer-to-peer interactions. Preschoolers have participated in LBT by participating in simple collaborative building activities—often with adult prompting—in simplified and supported versions of the basic triad model of part-supplier, engineer, and builder. The bricks are typically larger (for safety and fine motor skill reasons), and fewer per LEGO set, and the instructions are printed larger and with fewer steps. LEGO play activities can also involve non-building interactions such as racing pull-back cars, parallel play with stacking bricks or following simple brick patterns, sorting and sequencing bricks by color, size, and shape, etc.

The main goal of LBT with young learners is consistent with that for older children, which is to emphasize the social and cultural context of play and de-emphasize idiosyncratic sensory exploration or repetitive actions with the play materials. Learning to participate in the social communication and cultural context of play requires children to be responsive to and learn from the symbolic and representational features of play materials. In that sense, LEGO materials provide an excellent format for transitioning from object-play to toy-play, since LEGO bricks are both functional objects and symbolic representations. At some point in cognitive development, children acquire the capacity to shift from playing with toys as colorful or interesting objects, to experiencing them as transitional or symbolic representations with cultural meaning.

This is clear in the early learning materials available from LEGO but can also be emphasized in LBT activities at this developmental level.

This is an important role for LEGO therapists. Aside from facilitating the safe and non-intrusive physical proximity of the participants, therapists working with young LBT participants should be aware of the children's cognitive development needs within a constructivist framework. For preschool level LBT groups (developmental ages three to five years), there needs to be a lower participant-to-therapist ratio, around three-to-one, compared with early elementary school age children (developmental ages five to ten years) which can have a higher participant-to-therapist ratio of roughly six-to-one. Aside from simplifying the LEGO activities and including more adult involvement in them, choosing, and setting up the activities, implementing the LEGO level system, following LEGO rules, and using the "Rules of Cool," will all need to be communicated and implemented with increased adult input and support. Interactions and communication among group members will require more prompting from the therapists, although it is still important to emphasize peer-mediated input as much as possible. Rather than directly prompting or directing a child's actions in the whole LBT experience (from the time they arrived in the waiting room until they leave, or throughout the school-based activity), therapists should look for opportunities to prompt the children to communicate and interact with each other directly.

Advanced Learners in LBT. One of the most obvious divergent patterns of development in autistic children, aside from diminished sociality and identification with peers, is the difference between cognitive and social development. This is an observation that often leads the public and even some educational professionals to describe autistic children as having idiot savant qualities, also referred to in some publications as splinter skills. This is a common misconception which results from comparing the abilities and skills of autistic children with those of typically developing peers. The neurocognitive functioning of autistic children is not physiologically different from their peers with the exception that it is idiosyncratic and not organized by being integrated by their interest and participation in sociocultural systems. In other words, the cognitive abilities of autistic children can be normal, but the way they use those cognitive abilities is not.

The range of cognitive functioning among children with autism is as wide as it is in other populations of children, but what is not consistent are the sociocultural domains of cognitive functioning and this is evident from birth or even before birth. Ironically, the idea that an autistic child's cognitive functioning shows deficits, is uneven, or shows splinter skills, results from the anthropocentric bias of our developmental assessment procedures. Both the description of developmental benchmarks for perceptual-motor, social, language, cognitive, and academic domains (e.g., Vineland-3, ABAS-3, WIAT-4) and the tests used to assess these abilities directly, known as IQ tests (e.g., K-BIT, Stanford-Binet, WISC-5), were developed using observations and assessments of typical children, that is, anthropocentric children. Essentially what age-referenced measures of adaptive development like the Vineland-3 and ABAS-3 measure are evidence that a child is internalizing knowledge and skills that are meaningful and useful to those around them, not to the child themselves. In typical children, the child happens to identify with others, and is motivated to be like them, so they agree that they should be using their learning abilities to acquire skills that are necessary for participation in sociocultural systems. Autistic children may have the same sensory-perceptual, motor, and cognitive abilities, but their interests and aptitudes are guided by their own learning experiences, not those that are part of their sociocultural context.

Given that, there is a recognized subgroup of autistic children who have a combination of high cognitive abilities in terms of abstract reasoning, memory capacity, rate of learning, complex visualization, and problem-solving, yet have poor theory-of-mind, social reasoning and problem-solving, and deficits in age-typical capacity for peer relationships and social communication. The LBT approach to improving sociocultural adaptation seems to work especially well for this population. LEGO-based activities are a common play material for many or most children today (depending on national and cultural context, of course), but the opportunity to engage with a complex system which does not limit their creative ideas, willingness to address technical challenges, or their individual interests, is especially attractive for cognitively advanced children. In the LBT model, these children tend to thrive, but the challenge for the LEGO Club and therapists is to facilitate their participation in the group without unnecessarily frustrating or limiting that participation.

The LEGO level system offers group members the opportunity to advance quickly to the higher levels of Expert, Genius, and then Legend, based on their LEGO-based building and designing skills, but the levels also include social competency benchmarks. Many cognitive advanced children are initially ambitious and optimistic about getting to the higher LEGO levels quickly until they are faced with social collaboration and communication challenges. These group members are often likely to appeal to the therapist or other high-level group members to allow them to do more individual work and bypass the social-communication requirements.

It is important to emphasize to advanced learners early on that they need to meet the social-communication requirements of the level system. Doing so can be frustrating for them, but in the end, it can be extremely beneficial since they are likely to meet similar sorts of challenges later in their educational and vocational careers. Many young adults with high cognitive abilities but who have low sociality and poor social and communication skills end up either unemployed or under-employed despite their potential for creative participation in those systems. Although the child and even their parents may express frustration or irritation with a child feeling stuck as a LEGO Builder or Creator, they will certainly appreciate it later if they put in the work on social communication and collaboration skills if they legitimately achieve LEGO Expert and LEGO Genius at this stage. Their future adaptability and competency in sociocultural systems including employment will be worth the effort.

Integrating LBT with Developmental and Educational Goals. Although it is always good to have some informal level of communication with other developmental services agencies and school districts as a service provider, that involvement can also be more formal. Many of the children who participated in the original LEGO Club groups in Hawaii were referred for psychological and social development services by the state department of health (Hawaii's Child and Adolescent Mental Health Centers) or their school districts. As such, the LEGO Club and LBT were components of their health department individual family services plans (IFSPs), or their school's special education individualized education plans (IEPs). Those plans require the professional members of a child's IFSP or IEP team to submit pre-services assessment reports, service plans with goals and benchmarks for outcome monitoring, and treatment updates and discharge summaries. If a child's services plan continues for years, as many do, the professionals involved are also required to submit annual and triannual norm-referenced assessment reports.

As described previously, these forms of documentation were important to the history of the development of LBT as an evidence-based strategy since the outcome data for participants could be aggregated and meaningfully compared across participants because it included standardized and norm-referenced measures. In some private school and clinic settings there may not be a requirement for these sorts of structured assessments, treatment plans, or outcome measures, but there may still be requirements from parents and other stakeholders (and possibly public-school districts who are funding out-of-district services) for evidence of benefit. This is an area that has in recent years become dominated by behavior analytic influences which focus on short-term observable goals, and in fact, many health insurance carriers and school districts require behavioral objectives as a component of their utilization review and implementation standards.

It is essential for LBT therapists and educators not to fall into the trap of focusing on behaviorally defined objectives. The experimental analysis of behavior and behavioral objectives were developed initially using operant conditioning paradigms in animal laboratories (Skinner, 1966; Ferster, 1953; Skinner, 1938) before they were introduced into educational (Skinner, 1968) and developmental and clinical settings (Skinner, 1978; Ferster, 1961; Ferster & DeMyer, 1961). As has been described previously (LeGoff, 2023), the definition of behavior in operant conditioning paradigms was shaped by the methodology which was designed to allow researchers to collect automatically generated rates (frequencies over time) or durations of actions, which were both repeatable and amenable to extinction. In other words, they defined "behavior," in ways that supported the theory of operant conditioning. This was not a scientific goal, but a politically motivated one: Skinner wanted to prove that behavior could be controlled by its positive and negative consequences, and to demonstrate that, he focused his efforts on demonstrating this using small animals who would engage in discrete, repeatable behaviors like rats pressing a lever or pigeons pecking at a key which could be reinforced on specific schedules using automated food pellet dispensing equipment.

Those repeatable actions by small animals in operant conditioning chambers and the artificial food-pellet positive reinforcement may have nothing in common with human social learning, but that is not what Skinner and Ferster asserted. In fact, Skinner took the extra step of giving an elaborate theoretical description of how children's acquisition of language as a means of communication could have been due to natural versions of operant conditioning (Skinner, 1957). Despite being an untenable theory, based on the observed patterns of language and communication development in humans and other species (Chomsky, 1959; 1957), Ivar Lovaas and his followers initiated using the same sorts of laboratory methods developed by Skinner and Ferster, and as recommended by Skinner for educators. Skinner did not do research on human subjects, and he was not trained in child development, education, or clinical psychology, but the methods he outlined for making objective recordings of repeated discrete learning trials were convenient ways to record the compliance with learning drills and became widely popular after being introduced as a treatment for autism by Ferster (1961) and then by Lovaas and his colleagues (Lovaas, 1993; Lovaas, *et al*, 1974; 1973).

Although the studies by Lovaas which described intensive early interventions involving up to 40 hours per week of discrete trial sessions were not able to be replicated, the extension of Skinner and Ferster's discrete-trial definitions of how to objectively quantify observable and measurable rates of repeatable and reversible actions left an indelible impression on special education settings, especially those which served children with diverse developmental differences. Social and communication abilities in children have never been properly understood as behaviors, yet educational institutions to this day hold service provider responsible for quantitative descriptions of discrete actions as the benchmarks of educational or therapeutic benefit. What this approach for assessing outcomes ignores is that sociocultural adaptation involves qualitative changes in action, not quantitative ones, and the more important outcomes have to do with how a child participates in a system, not the rate or duration of an observed action. It is not as important how often or for how long a child does something, it is important how those actions are experienced by others and that child as being relevant and helpful to a shared system that is maintained by collaborative contributions.

In that context, what was written earlier about using outcome measures which reflect social adjustment and adaptability overall is more important and relevant to the goals of education. Behavioral objectives are necessarily quantitative (number, frequency, rate, duration), and their model (operant conditioning) is simply not compatible with understanding either the internal (constructivist), or the external (social constructivist) systems involved. That does not mean that treatment outcomes cannot be written as objectives with operationalized benchmarks. It means that those benchmarks should not be defined by quantitative measures or methods derived from operant conditioning paradigms. Parent and teacher ratings of social adjustment, as well as standardized measures of sociality (e.g., SSRS or Vineland-3 Socialization Domain), and observations of peer-based activities (e.g., mean duration of social interaction with peers during free play), and peer-to-peer social ratings in classrooms, are all objective measures which are not derived from operant conditioning methods.

Facilitating peer mediation, conflict resolution, and collaboration, not adult direction. There is no doubt that interpersonal problems and miscommunication will arise in LEGO Club. The limited availability of time and materials, the close physical proximity, and the fact that the members are pre-selected to having poor social skills guarantee that collaborative LEGO building is not going to occur without some interpersonal conflicts. Some of the more acute (and hilarious) problems can result from group members being exposed to negative forms of social communication and interaction in their homes, schools, and communities, and then imitatively trying them out in LEGO Club. Teasing and bullying are not natural interpersonal actions for autistic children, but they will be exposed to these situations with their siblings, extended family, or peers. Sexualized and other forms of aggressive or inappropriate humor can also be picked up and then tried out in LEGO Club.

One of the most important rules for LBT therapists is not to get caught up in the excitement (autonomic arousal) that can be quickly generated in these situations. Becoming more assertive, louder, or initiating threats about exclusion, getting parents involved, or other disciplinary actions is invariably ineffective or counterproductive. Group dynamics can quickly turn from synergistic to neutral (stalled) or negative (antergistic) if the therapist(s) joins the conflict and excitement rather than following a proactive or preventative plan of action. Therapists who use their adult voices to shout, or their adult authority to threaten, are ignoring the fact that the group members will not necessarily understand why that is acceptable as a coping strategy for the therapist, but not for them. The LEGO Club rules are intended for the group members, not the therapist, but that presumes that the therapist does not start acting like a group member and joining in arguments and disputes.

Negative interactions between group members can occur and escalate quickly, so the best approach is not to rely on consequences, but to plan and set up events for the group activities which avoid interpersonal flashpoints. This means that group members should not enter the LEGO Club waiting room when they are already worked up and violating social norms or being oppositional with their parents. Having parents on board with this is important, but that needs to be communicated to the children as well: they will not be allowed to enter the clinic's waiting room, let alone the LEGO Club, if they are overly excited and being disruptive. Parents can be given a simple directive to make sure that a child is calm enough to follow verbal directions from home to the vehicle, etc., and they can check for signs of over-arousal like sweating, excessive motor activity, disinhibited speech, or a heart rate of over 100 beats per minute.

This can be difficult for parents who are running late for LEGO Club, which by itself can result in frustration and over-arousal, which then exacerbates the issue of having to calm down before being allowed into the group. Teaching group members and their parents how to use mental imagery or three slow breaths to decrease autonomic arousal, or progressive muscle relaxation (PMR), and to do this before each group, is a good strategy. This can also be carried over to the group sessions, especially if a group member or multiple group members have gotten close to being out of control during group sessions, by having group members start out by doing deep breathing or PMR during the check-in and planning phase. Normally, though, just participating in the focused discussion about the previous week's activities and the planning for the current session offers an opportunity for group members to become calm and focused.

Aside from using the peer-mentors to function as intermediaries in group member disputes (described below), there are two anticipatory strategies which can be used in the absence of input from peer mentors. The first approach involves steering the attention of group members away from conflicts or disruptive acting towards other ongoing actions which are either incompatible with or not part of the conflict. For example, not responding to a conflict between two members about how to solve a LEGO building problem, or whose turn it is to perform a certain task, and instead commenting on the collaborative actions of another pair or whatever the rest of the group members are engaged in. Reinterpreting or reframing conflicts can also be helpful, for instance by commenting on how motivated and diligent group members are, which is evident in their motivation to participate. A group member being self-centered or wanting to take more than their share of the resources or the group time can be reframed as being motivated to contribute their efforts.

Another effective strategy is to prescribe prosocial or helpful actions in a way which capitalizes on an otherwise selfish motive, and then relabeling the compliance as generosity. A group member who may be engaged in an individual activity not involving the group, for example, could be asked to continue their activity as a way of helping the group with another activity. Or they might be asked to describe for the other group members what they are working on as a way of instructing other group members. Complimenting group members for their LEGO-based skills can be a successful way of then transitioning from that compliment to getting the other group members to request their support and involvement. "Look at Aaron working on his free-style project, guys. He's very good at freestyle building, alright. Does anyone think Aaron might be able to help build something for the movie set? Pauline, can you ask Aaron if he would be willing build something for the movie set?"

Shared experience: Learning about life and development from each other. When the LEGO Club activities are underway and the group members are interacting and communicating efficiently with each other, they often can become routine. Like many work settings, co-workers can continue their assigned tasks and even communicate and collaborate while still being able to interact in more social ways and about more personal topics. This informal and more personal level of communication often happens in the waiting room, and at the beginning of LEGO Club sessions, where the group members are less actively engaged in projects. This is like the sort of informal social communication that happens during breaks at work, or when co-workers spend time together after work. Although communication and interaction among co-workers at these times is not considered part of their job duties, they are nonetheless an important part of what most people expect from work relationships. This can be a painful discovery for parents when they become aware that their otherwise intelligent, talented, and creative adult child has become isolated and depressed, stuck at a workstation, and not socializing with co-workers, and not receiving appropriate promotions.

That is one of the reasons that LEGO therapists are encouraged to take an active interest in not only what is going on in the waiting room before and after group sessions, but also to keep up with individual members and their families about personal life experiences at home and at school. While those are not necessarily going to be addressed effectively through the LBT process, they are "grist for the mill," when it comes to informal interpersonal disclosure and sharing of personal experiences. Getting peer feedback about ongoing issues, like conflicts with siblings or classmates, or struggling with complex social nuances, or even just modeling how other children engage in interpersonal chats, is just as important to the LBT process as the LEGO activities. For some group members, just knowing that another group member has parents, siblings, pets, a home, and interests and hobbies outside of LEGO Club can be an improvement in their social competence. They begin to get a sense of the degrees of freedom or variables of other people's social lives: the other people, their relationships, conflicts, modes of communication, and cultural experiences. Children with autism are often unaware of many of the standard set of social questions and they do not yet understand why other people might be interested in their relationships, preferences, and activities.

Part of the benefit of participating in LEGO Club is that it exposes the members to other children with whom they can identify. As was said by one of the first members of the first LEGO Club, "Dr. Dan, that kid if from my planet." The interest in each other, the experience of having at least one shared value—LEGO—and the feeling of identifying yourself with others (they are like me), create the basis for having more than just a working relationship during the group sessions. That social identification motivates children to want to know more about each other and to share about themselves. For the average eight- or ten-year-old child, sharing personal information does not come naturally, but typical children are still aware of how adults engage in social banter and sharing of personal information, and soon they are able to model their parents and other adults' styles of social communication. The learning curve for this activity is much steeper for autistic children who are discovering that other children are like them for the first time, and they are not intuitively able to model social nuances and norms. They do not have an internalized sense of what is appropriate to disclose when, how to use humor to diffuse tension in emotional situations, or how to disclose in reciprocal ways.

There are many age and gender-related norms in this regard. Girls tend to disclose more than boys, and older children disclose more than younger children. There are also norms about certain topics, which most older children and adults understand intuitively are personal or "taboo," such as toileting, personal health issues, personal finances, race, and religion. Strongly emotional topics can be shared by group members who have established relationships, but those can take a while to develop, and more superficial topics are usually safer for acquaintances or those who have not shared much about their personal lives so far. These invisible norms of personal disclosure, asking for help from others, and asking personal questions can all be commented on or given subtle direction from the therapist. Preferably, though, these are opportunities for the more senior group members, and certainly the LEGO

Legend peer mentors to get involved. Although they may not understand that this is part of their role—they often think of themselves as LEGO experts, not personal advisors, or life coaches—in my experience they are invariably helpful when asked by the therapist to become more actively involved.

Understanding play and culture: Transgenerational knowledge, skills, and creativity. Knowledge and understanding are like other abilities and skills in that they may not always be based on individual experience or even on a child's conscious awareness. This is referred to in neuropsychology as the difference between declarative information (knowing that we know something) and procedural information or skills (knowing how to do something). Children are born with abilities which allow them to develop knowledge, understanding, and skills through a variety of experiences, some of which are involve simple, direct experiences, some involve social learning through modeling and imitation, and others involve various forms of communication. Learning how to build and create with LEGO, for instance, often starts with a child's direct manipulation of LEGO bricks and putting them together in various ways. Their level of knowledge, understanding, and skill will be limited, however, without the addition of the scaffolding effect of models, such as watching older siblings, peers, or adults engage with those materials in more elaborate and innovative ways. That is what Bruner called scaffolding, and it is responsible for what Vygotsky called the zone of proximal difference—the difference between what a child can learn based on their own abilities, and what they are able to achieve with the help of parents, teachers, and mentors. Finally, children learn even more about the uses and creative potential for LEGO by watching YouTube videos, reading books about LEGO, or watching documentaries, TV shows, or other media sources on the topic.

These sources of learning through experience, modeling, and communication are how many therapists and educators think about the passing down of culture and knowledge from one generation to the next. What is missing from that view, however, is the reciprocal process by which children who are learning and developing their skills contribute back to their social and cultural systems. If learning and culture was simply a unidirectional process, an informational one-way street from one generation to the next, culture would change very slowly if at all. What is important about culture, like any other dynamic complex system, is that it must not become rigid and therefore cannot rely on occasional random mistakes to create the diversity of actions that is necessary for adaptive flexibility.

Genes and culture both benefit from randomness at times, as well as more systematic forms of change, such as mating processes. Animals choose mates based on observed behavioral and physical characteristics, which influences the characteristics and adaptive fitness of their offspring. Culture benefits from occasional accidents, but more importantly, humans are generally not content to do exactly what their parents did. They learn how to use the technologies, language, and social systems of their culture as they exist—whether that is in a small village in the middle of nowhere, or in a densely populated city—and then play with it.

Becoming proficient with the knowledge, skills, technology, social norms, and modes of communication of a child's culture has three important results other than improving that child's adaptability: first, it identifies that child are part of that culture and highlights for the adults in that culture the value that has now been invested in the child in terms of the sustainability of their culture: "They're one of us now." Second, being "one of us," does not imply only a social identity, a sense of belonging, it also implies the successful persistence of cultural values and the reassurance that for at least another generation or two, that sociocultural system and those values will continue. Finally, because children acquire sociocultural knowledge and skills in ways that involve play, adults are especially gratified or reassured when they observe that their children are playing in culturally specific ways. That means that not only are children "one of us," and that they will continue the traditions and values of their ancestors, but that they will do so in creative ways. In other words, their culture will continue in adaptive ways.

That is why learning and development is not just acquiring new information or skills in various ways. If culture is to continue to survive, it must be adaptable, and for it to be adaptable, it must be flexible, it must be capable of generating innovations, or creating entirely new degrees of freedom through creativity. The viability of any sociocultural system, then, relies on one of the most natural and underestimated forms of learning: play. Parents, teachers, therapists, and other adults in any society do not insist that their children play in exactly the ways that they did, although they do like to see some consistency between the activities and materials they had as children are also part of today's play. We become intuitively anxious about rapid, large changes in play activities which can come from de novo play products coming on the market—like all the recent technologically sophisticated toys and games—or from other cultures or societies. Some degree of change in play patterns of the next generation is reassuring and expected, but too much is anxiety-provoking for the previous generations.

LEGO is happily one of those play materials which has both a sense of stability over time—a lot of adults still play with LEGO, and they seem to especially enjoy collecting and building with LEGO materials that remind them of their own childhood experiences—and flexibility through innovation and creative ideas. The LEGO materials of today have both completely novel applications—like video games, and programmable robotics—as well as many familiar and traditional elements, like the venerable LEGO City and LEGO Creator series, and the old sets that are still for sale on Bricklink.com. Soon enough, LBT and LEGO Club will be in their second generation, and that is one of the reasons this manual is written without a lot of specific information about how to run LBT or LEGO Clubs. These have always been and should remain organic processes that have a stable sense of identity and boundary around what is or is not part of LEGO Club, but the process should also remain open to playful interpretation and creative adaptability. If LBT is a strategy for exposing children to a microcosm of sociocultural systems in the form of the LEGO Club, it must continue to be not just a playful and creative process for the participants, but a playful and creative process for those who facilitate it.

Common mistakes in setting up and facilitating LEGO Club groups. Since starting the first LBT group in the late 1990's, I have been involved in initiating dozens of my own groups in different states, using different formats, and in different institutional settings, some of which I have facilitated with other providers. There have also been opportunities for me to train and supervise the implementation of LEGO Club groups facilitated by other developmental specialists, therapists, and educators in the US and in many other countries. By far the largest number of active LBT groups has been in the UK, largely thanks to the work of Dr. Gina Gomez de la Cuesta (nee Owens), who did the first independent replication study of LBT (Owens, *et al*, 2008), and her colleague, Dr. Elinor Brett (Brett, 2013), who also completed independent outcome research on LBT. In addition to the efforts of their group, *Play Included*, there have been several professionals who have been involved in both facilitating LEGO Club groups as well as training and supervising other therapists in South and Central America, Europe, Australia, and New Zealand, and both Central and Southeast Asia.

Although most of the LEGO Club groups I have observed are being implemented with integrity to the model, and often with considerable creativity and resourcefulness required by less than ideal physical and financial conditions. Based on having learned from my own numerous missteps and poor judgment, as well as the evidence from some LBT groups that seemed to be less effective than they might have been, I would like to offer some recommendations about avoiding some strategies or ways of thinking about LEGO Club that are not consistent with the overall model, and therefore may detract from the benefit of it.

- Primarily, LEGO Club is a child-led and peer-mediated intervention. It is not based on applications of ABA (operant conditioning), naturalistic or otherwise, and is not intended to teach children how to play with LEGO. As should be clear by now, the goal of LBT is to create a therapeutic environment which allows children to experience the benefits of being part of peer-group collaborations. Top-down adult direction interferes with the dynamics of both peer-to-peer, group-to-child, and child-to-group collaborations and synergistic outcomes. Setting up LEGO Club groups and facilitating them needs to be done in ways which are unobtrusive and do not interfere with the peer group dynamics.
- The peer-group synergy in LEGO Club can also be interfered with by having other professionals who do not understand how LBT works get involved, or by having parents attend the sessions with their children. While it is possible for other professionals, or mentors, and possibly even parents or siblings to attend or even lead a LEGO Club group, they need to understand the operational dynamics, individual and group goals, and the unobtrusive facilitation processes. Most of the time, non-group members and non-LBT-trained facilitators will have their own interests or goals for being involved, and those can interfere with the synergy and positive peer-group experience of LEGO Club.
- Teaching children how to play is unnecessary. All children play, and in fact, all mammalian offspring play. There are many forms of play which involve LEGO materials, and a child's interest and skill level with LEGO may be limiting factors for participating with peers who may be more advanced in their LEGO skills, but that is not something that the therapist should be addressing in the LEGO Club group session. If a child has perceptual-motor coordination or motor planning difficulties which

limit their LEGO-based skill acquisition, they may benefit from individual occupational therapy, or one-on-one LEGO-based therapy sessions before joining a LEGO Club. If a child joins a LEGO Club group and is struggling to achieve the basic helper skills, the other group members should be enlisted to model, support, and coach them, but the therapist should use this as an opportunity to facilitate the investment of the other group members in helping that child to become a contributor to their collaborative efforts, not simply direct or teach a group member. That dynamic results in isolating the child from their peers, not enhancing their opportunity to participate.

- The use of the diagnostic term, Autism Spectrum Disorder (ASD), has become so widely used for such a range of developmental, psychosocial, and self-regulation conditions that it has become virtually meaningless. The Centers for Disease Control in the US estimated recently that ASD is being diagnosed in one out of every thirty-six children. That rate has been growing steadily for the past couple of decades, but especially since the revision of the DSM-5 criteria which replaced the entire category of Pervasive Developmental Disorders with ASD. It is not recommended that participants in LBT be selected based on having been diagnosed with ASD. Many children with that diagnosis have nothing in common other than that label. Including children in LBT should be based on more careful assessment of their needs, and of the likelihood that they will be able to identify with, collaborate with, and experience a sense of shared identity, shared accomplishment, and mutual benefit from the LEGO Club experience.

- The room, furniture, and materials in LEGO Club groups should facilitate the overall experience of a peer-based activity, not the convenience of the adult therapists or observers. The facilitators of LBT need to pay attention to the sensory qualities of the room including the lighting, furnishings, room dimensions, and sound quality. Windows which are open to the outside which allow visual or auditory distractions can be a problem. The air temperature should be appropriate for the size and proximity of the children. The furniture should also be developmentally and socially appropriate for the group members. As mentioned above, ensure there is adequate space and furniture in the waiting room and restroom facilities. The space should not be cluttered and busy with other materials or contain potentially distracting electronic devices. The LEGO Club activities should also have an appropriate physical boundary, not just an area or table in an otherwise actively occupied room.

- It is reasonable and expected that group members will want to share their own LEGO projects with the other group members, but as mentioned earlier, have them share via social media or by bringing photos or cell-phone pictures. That sharing should be done in the waiting room, unless otherwise approved by the therapist/facilitator and other group leaders: bringing cell phones or other electronic devices, LEGO materials, or non-LEGO play materials can be distracting and lead to conflicts. If a group member has brought something to share with the group—whether it is a LEGO book, or cookies, or birthday cake, or a graduation diploma—they should ask the other group members and the facilitator if they can bring it into the LEGO Club. Keep in mind that the semi-permeable boundary of the LEGO Club system is maintained by the group, not individual members, or their parents.

- Allowing siblings or other non-client peers to participate in LBT can be problematic for a variety of reasons. One of the most common problems that results from outsiders attending is that they may take a lot of attention away from group members, not necessarily by being disruptive, but by being having better LEGO-based and social-communication skills than the group members. When a group member rises through the LEGO level system and graduates to become a LEGO Legend and peer mentor, the other group members can identify with them as "like me," and a model for them; an example to strive towards. A group member's brother or sister, or friend, or classmate from school who is well-behaved, friendly, and very good at LEGO might be a good LBT mentor, but they might also just make the other group members feel inadequate and feel that their special place where they can be themselves and feel good about having peers who accept them and identify with them, has been invaded by one of the "them." The sense of "us," in LEGO Club needs to be protected. If a non-member is introduced as a mentor, they should clearly be older or otherwise identified as a mentor, otherwise they can threaten the sense of "us," and disrupt the experience of group cohesion and synergy.

LEGO Club and LBT are not based on or consistent with "sensory integration," or multisensory learning models. The group activities need to be based on the interaction of the group members with LEGO play materials.

It is a form of group play therapy and does not have behavioral or sensory objectives. The activities, methods, and benefits of LBT need to be focused on, and documented consistent with the LBT model. That model is based on the theory and research which indicates that some children are lower on trait sociality than others simply because of normal variability in the population distribution of that trait. The consequences of lower sociality or the BAP can include having features of ASD which are described in the DSM-5 (American Psychiatric Association, 2013), or autistic disorder, Asperger's disorder, or atypical autism, as described in the ICD-10 (World Health Organization, 2019). Those conditions reflect what has been described here and elsewhere (LeGoff, 2023), as a multifactorial maladaptive antergistic outcome. Antergy in that sense, is the opposite of the adaptive and creative influence of synergistic dynamics: rather than working together to support successful adaptation, the contributing elements of an antergistic system work against adaptability, resulting in persistent and predictable failures to adapt, or maladaptive outcomes.

The goal of LBT, then, is to prevent or reverse the maladaptive influences of factors like social withdrawal and isolation, interpersonal hostility and rejection, lack of identity with peers, poor self-efficacy, social anxiety, pessimism, low self-esteem, feelings of helplessness, hopelessness, depressed mood, anger and irritability, psychological reactance, and sociocultural learning difficulties, all of which can be the negative and complex, complementary or exacerbating results of life experiences which follow from low trait sociality or BAP. When describing or communicating about LBT, it is important to reference this model, and not to confuse or obscure the LBT model with incompatible theories or methods.

CONCLUSION

LEGO-based therapy is a promising form of social development therapy and psychosocial adjustment therapy which has been used in therapy clinics and schools for over twenty years. There is a growing body of evidence regarding the methods and benefits, primarily for children with autistic conditions. It is also generally accepted clinically that LBT is an effective strategy for children with internalizing conditions (anxiety, depressed mood, social adjustment difficulties), but there has not been outcome research published using other non-autistic populations. The current manuscript provides an update and expands discussion of the research evidence and theoretic framework for LBT following the publication of the first outcome studies (Owens, *et al*, 2008; LeGoff & Sherman, 2006; LeGoff, 2004), and the first LBT treatment manual (LeGoff, *et al*, 2014). This manuscript emphasizes the theoretical model for LBT as being influenced by the social constructivist model of Vygotsky (1933), general systems theory of Ludwig von Bertalanffy (1950), the synergistic degrees of freedom approach to movement studies by Nikolai Bernstein (1967) and Mark Latash (2008), and the evolutionary systems theory of Peter Corning (2018). The model is also derived and supported by the theories and research on the sociocultural value of play in both child development and human evolution (Muthukrishna, *et al*, 2018; Burghardt, 2015; LaFreniere, 2011; Goncu & Gaskins, 2006; Goncu, 1999), the evidence of innate sociality in typical infant development (Meltzoff, *et al*, 2009), and the central role of sociality on typical child development and sociocultural systems (Grandvist, 2021; Pinker, 2010; Tomasello, *et al*, 2005).

The current model views LBT as offering children with low sociality—defined as a normal but low level of anthropocentrism (a natural bias towards environmental events involving people and their stuff)—which can result in difficulties with adapting to sociocultural systems. Since children are expected to be able to acquire knowledge and skills at typical rates using sociocultural supports (parents, siblings, classrooms), children who are less interested in these systems are at a disadvantage in terms of benefiting from and contributing to sociocultural systems, including education and employment. The LBT model creates a microcosm of these other sociocultural systems by utilizing the shared interest that many autistic children have for LEGO and supporting their positive experience as members of a LEGO Club. The LBT therapist facilitates collaborative activities, and interpersonal communication, in ways that reflect other forms of interpersonal collaboration in sociocultural settings, emphasizing the benefits of interpersonal and group synergy, and creative play. This model is consistent with what we know about how typical children can develop social and cultural knowledge and skills through play.

Based on direct observation of autistic children who participate in LBT, it is immediately apparent that they have a favorable response to the LEGO Club, including the opportunity to participate with peers in LEGO-based construction activities and creative play. What has also been obvious for some time is that children who have fun and engage in playful activities such as LEGO Club are motivated to continue their involvement, and to expand that experience to include other children in other settings (LeGoff & Sherman, 2006; LeGoff, 2004). What is sometimes obscured by autism intervention strategies which emphasize short-term observable behavioral outcomes—ABA-based interventions—is that neither play nor child development can be meaningfully accounted for as operant behaviors. Most of what children need to learn to participate in modern societies involve learning how to communicate, use technology, and maintain relationships with other people in ways that most children learn by participating in sociocultural systems. Culture and society themselves are emergent systems of social synergy: people working together for their mutual benefit and that of their social groups.

Longer term adaptive outcomes for children and young adults who are born less inclined to identify with others and to collaborate with them is not improved by using external rewards (reinforcers) to encourage them to increase rates of target behaviors. Children low on sociality—whether they are classified as autistic or not—will improve their sociocultural adjustment, including improving their communication, social interactions, and culturally-relevant technical skills if they have positive experiences of other children and sociocultural systems. Whitehouse, *et al* (2021) and Green, *et al* (2022), have shown the benefit of enhancing social play experiences in infants at risk for the BAP and autism using a brief and cost-effective parent-training model. LEGO Club is also a cost-effective, natural, and non-invasive model which increases the positive social play experiences of autistic and at-risk children and adolescents. Unfortunately, neither of these approaches has received the level of higher-level administrative support or funding that has been offered to much more costly and invasive procedures based on ABA models, largely due to the marketing of ABA-based interventions as being synonymous with "evidence-based."

As has been described elsewhere (LeGoff, 2023), "evidence-based," should be interpreted to mean evidence of benefit consistent with scientific evidence, and not, "We have lots of evidence to justify what we are doing." As David Hume's *is-ought* distinction demonstrates, factual arguments cannot logically be used to justify moral or ethical decision-making. The negative experiences of children and their families in ABA-based programs is not now somehow reversed by "naturalistic" strategies which use ABA in less austere and punishing ways. The theoretical model that ABA is based on—operant conditioning—is a way of thinking about children that would be abhorrent to parents and educators alike if they took the time to read and understand it. Aside from not being morally justifiable as a model of child development, ABA is also not consistent with current scientific models of child development, neuroscience, or sociocultural systems. In that sense, ABA *is not* scientifically supportable, and *ought not* be promoted as a way of helping children learn and develop from a moral point of view.

In addition to the scientific concerns about the evidence regarding ABA's methods and outcomes, and the moral and ethical concerns about using this model as a form of education and therapy for human children, the public is being inundated with distorted media representations of ASD and its possible biological or genetic bases. The inflated epidemiological data and scare tactics about lifelong disability are fueling the growth of poorly regulated health and dietary supplements, unhealthy eating restrictions, sensory-integration and other questionable physiological treatments for children who may or may not have autism. The bigger issue of what the public media and both educational and healthcare administrators are referring to when they cite epidemiological and outcome research on "autism," is a topic for another book.

For the present book, if we accept that being autistic is a condition that more children are experiencing more often, and that it reflects some underlying difficulty with having positive life experiences with other children and learning how to adapt to complex sociocultural systems, then yes, being autistic is a growing problem. That problem needs to be understood, however, from both the point of view of educators and therapists as well as from that of the children who are experiencing it. Being autistic is not a childhood disorder, it is a problem that affects the relationship between some children and their sociocultural context. We hope that sociocultural systems eventually will adapt to the needs of diversely developing children and adults, including those who are not sold on the value of participating in those systems. For now, though, it may be helpful to offer children experiences which allow them to discover how sociocultural systems work and how they can be beneficial to them. In doing so, those systems will also be influenced in beneficial and adaptive ways. Both of those outcomes—the benefit for the individual and their sociocultural systems—is what LEGO-based therapy is designed to offer.

REFERENCES

Adolphs, R. & Tranel, D. (2000). Emotion recognition and the human amygdala. In, J. Eggleton, (Ed), *The amygdala, 2nd edition*. New York, NY: Oxford University Press, pp. 587–630.

Alessandro, C., Delis, I., Nori, F., Panzeri, S. & Berret, B. (2013). Muscle synergies in neuroscience and robotics: From input-space to task-space perspectives. *Frontiers in Computational Neuroscience, 7*, e43.

American Psychiatric Association (2013). *Diagnostic and Statistical Manual of Mental Disorders, Fifth Edition (DSM-5)*. Washington, DC: APA Press.

Anderson, K.A., Shattuck, P.T., Cooper, B.C., Roux, A.M. & Wagner, M. (2014). Prevalence and correlates of postsecondary residential status among young adults with an autism spectrum disorder. *Autism, 18*, 562–570.

Andras, M. (2012). The value of LEGO® Therapy in promoting social interaction in primary-aged children with autism. *Good Autism Practice, 13* (2), 18–25.

Andrews, D.S., Aksman, L., Kerns, C.M., Lee, J.K., *et al.* (2022). Association of amygdala development with different forms of anxiety in autism spectrum disorder. *Biological Psychiatry, 91* (11), 977–987.

Arsalidou, M. & Pascual-Leone, J. (2016). Constructivist developmental theory is needed in developmental neuroscience. *NPJ: Science of Learning, 1*, 16016.

Araujo, D. & Davids, K. (2011). What exactly is acquired during skill acquisition? *Journal of Consciousness Studies, 18* (3–4), 7–23.

Araujo, D. & Davids, K. (2016). Team synergies in sport: Theory and measures. *Frontiers in Psychology, 7*, e01449.

Arsenio, W.F., Adams, E. & Gold, J. (2009). Social information processing, moral reasoning, and emotion attributions: Relations with adolescents' reactive and proactive aggression. *Child Development, 80*, 1739–1755.

Ashmawi, N.S. & Hammoda, M.A. (2022). Early prediction and evaluation of risk of autism spectrum disorders. *Cureus, 14* (3), e23465.

Ashwin, C., Baron-Cohen, S., Wheelwright, S., O'Riordan, M. & Bullmore, E.T. (2007). Differential activation of the amygdala and the 'social brain' during fearful face processing in Asperger Syndrome. *Neuropsychologia, 45*, 2–14.

Baldwin, S., Costley, D. & Warren, A. (2014). Employment activities and experiences of adults with high- functioning autism and Asperger's disorder. *Journal of Autism and Developmental Disorders, 44* (10), 2440–2449.

Banerjee, A., Luong, J.A., Ho, A., Saib, A.O. & Ploski, J.E. (2016). Overexpression of Homer1a in the basal and lateral amygdala impairs fear conditioning and induces an autism-like social impairment. *Molecular Autism, 7*, e16.

Barakova, E., Bajracharya, P., Willemsen, M., Lourens, T. & Huskens, B. (2015). Long-term LEGO-based therapy with humanoid robot for children with ASD. *Expert Systems Journal of Knowledge, 32*, 698–709.

Baron Cohen, S. (2011). *The science of evil: On empathy and the origins of cruelty.* New York, NY: Basic Books.

Baron Cohen, S., Ring, H.A., Bullmore, E.T., Wheelwright, S., Ashwin, C. & Williams, S.C.R. (2000). The amygdala theory of autism. *Neuroscience and Biobehavioral Reviews, 24*, 355–364.

Bernaerts, S., Boets, B., Steyaert, J., *et al.* (2020). Oxytocin treatment attenuates amygdala activity in autism: A treatment-mechanism study with long-term follow-up. *Translational Psychiatry, 10*, e383.

Bernstein, N.A. (1926/2020). *Biomechanics for instructors.* R. Whyman (Trans). Cham, Switzerland: Springer Nature.

Bernstein, N.A. (1947/2020). *On the construction of movements: The original text and commentaries.* M.L. Latash, (Ed. & translator). New York, NY: Routledge Publishing.

Bernstein, N.A. (1948/1996). On dexterity and its development. In, M.L. Latash & M.T. Turvey (Eds.), *Dexterity and its development.* Hillsdale, NJ: Lawrence Erlbaum Associates, pp. 1–235.

Bernstein, N.A. (1967). *The coordination and regulation of movements.* Oxford, UK: Pergamon Press.

Bettelheim, B. (1967). *The empty fortress: Infantile autism and the birth of the self.* New York, NY: The Free Press.

Boyne, S.E.J. (2014). *An evaluation of the 'LEGO® Therapy' intervention used to support children with social communication difficulties in their mainstream classroom.* Doctoral thesis in educational psychology, University of Nottingham, Nottingham, UK.

Brehm, J.W. (1966). *A theory of psychological reactance.* New York, NY: Academic Press.

Brehm, J.W. & Brehm, S.S. (1981). *Psychological reactance: A theory of freedom and control.* New York, NY: Academic Press.

Brehm, J.W. (1993). Control, its loss, and psychological reactance. In, G. Weary, F. Gleicher, & K.L. Marsh (Eds.), *Control motivation and social cognition.* Geneva, SU: Springer Verlag.

Brehm, J.W. & Cohen, A.R. (1962). *Explorations in cognitive dissonance.* New York: Wiley.

Brett, E. (2013). *LEGO Therapy: Developing social competence in children with Asperger syndrome through collaborative LEGO play.* Doctoral Thesis in educational child and community psychology, University of Exeter, Exeter, UK.

Brody, H. (1973). The systems view of man: Implications for medicine, science, and ethics. *Perspectives in Biology and Medicine, 17* (1), 71–92.

Brooks, R. & Meltzoff, A.N. (2015). Connecting the dots from infancy to childhood: A longitudinal study connecting gaze following, language, and explicit theory of mind. *Journal of Experimental Child Psychology, 130,* 67–78.

Bruner, J.S. (1973). *The relevance of education.* New York, NY: Norton.

Bruner, J.S. (1979). *On knowing: Essays for the left hand.* Cambridge, MS: Harvard University Press.

Bruner, J.S. (1986). *Actual minds, possible worlds.* Cambridge, MS: Harvard University Press.

Burghardt, G.M. (2015). Creativity, play, and the pace of evolution. In, A. B. Kaufman & J. C. Kaufman (Eds.), *Animal creativity and innovation.* Baltimore, MD: Elsevier Academic Press (pp. 129–161).

Cage, E., Di Monaco, J. & Newell, V. (2018). Experiences of autism acceptance and mental health in autistic adults. *Journal of Autism and Developmental Disorders, 48* (2), 473–484.

Cage, E. & Troxell-Whitman, Z. (2019). Understanding the reasons, contexts and costs of camouflaging for autistic adults. *Journal of Autism and Developmental Disorders, 49* (5), 1899–1911.

Chamak, B. & Bonniau, B. (2016). Trajectories, long-term outcomes and family experiences of 76 adults with autism spectrum disorder. *Journal of Autism and Developmental Disorders, 46* (3), 1084–1095.

Chapman, R. (2021). Neurodiversity and the social ecology of mental functions. *Perspectives on Psychological Science, 16* (6), 1360–1372.

Chamak, B. & Bonniau, B., (2016). Trajectories, long-term outcomes and family experiences of 76 adults with autism spectrum disorder. *Journal of Autism and Developmental Disorders, 46* (3), 1084–1095.

Chamberlain, P. (2017). Toward creating synergy among policy, procedures, and implementation of evidence-based models in child welfare systems: Two case examples. *Clinical Child and Family Psychology Review, 20* (1), 78–86.

Chau, L.S. & Galvez, R. (2012). Amygdala's involvement in facilitating associative learning-induced plasticity: A promiscuous role for the amygdala in memory acquisition. *Frontiers in Integrative Neuroscience, 6*, e0092.

Cheng, Y.F.S. (2016). *The effectiveness of the LEGO therapy intervention in promoting the social interaction of children with autism spectrum condition on the playground: An evaluation study*. Doctoral thesis in educational child and adolescent psychology, University College London, London, UK.

Chomsky, N. (1957). *Syntactic structures*. Berlin, FDR: Walter de Gruyter.

Chomsky, N. (1959). A review of B.F. Skinner's *Verbal Behavior. Language, 35* (1), 26–58.

Corning, P.A. (2003). *Nature's magic: Synergy in evolution and the fate of humankind*. New York: Cambridge University Press.

Corning, P.A. (2005). *Holistic Darwinism: Synergy, cybernetics, and the bioeconomics of evolution*. Chicago: University of Chicago Press.

Corning, P.A. (2011). *The fair society: The science of human nature and the pursuit of social justice*. Chicago, IL: University of Chicago Press.

Corning, P.A. (2018). *Synergistic selection: How cooperation has shaped evolution and the rise of humankind*. Hackensack, NJ: World Scientific Publishing.

Corning, P. (2022). A systems theory of biological evolution. *Biosystems, 214*, e104630.

Courchesne, E., Gazestani, V.H. & Lewis, N.E. (2020). Prenatal origins of ASD: The when, what and how of ASD development. *Trends in Neuroscience, 43* (5), 326–342.

Crawford, P.D. (2010). Educating for moral ability: Reflections on moral development based on Vygotsky's theory of concept formation. *Journal of Moral Education, 30* (2), 113–129.

Creanza, N., Kolodny, O. & Feldman, M.W. (2017). Cultural evolutionary theory: How culture evolves and why it matters. *Proceedings of the National Academy of Sciences of the United States of America, 114* (30), 7782–7789.

Crowell, J.A., Keluskar, J. & Gorecki, A. (2019). Parenting behavior and the development of children with autism spectrum disorder. *Comprehensive Psychiatry, 90*, 21–29.

Curseu, P.L., Meslec, N., Pluut, H. & Lucas, G.J.M. (2015). Cognitive synergy in groups and group-to-individual transfer of decision-making competencies. *Frontiers in Psychology, 6*, e1375.

Davis, R. & Crompton, C.J. (2021). What do new findings about social interaction in autistic adults mean for neurodevelopmental research? *Perspectives on Psychological Science: A Journal of the Association for Psychological Science, 16* (3), 649–653.

Dawson, G., Toth, K., Abbott, R., Osterling, J., Munson, J. & Estes, A. (2004). Early social attention impairments in autism: Social orienting, joint attention, and attention to distress. *Developmental Psychology, 40*, 271-283.

de Boer, B. (2017). Evolution of speech and evolution of language. *Psychonomic Bulletin & Review, 24*, 158–162.

Decety, J. (2020, Ed.). *The social brain: A developmental perspective.* Boston, MA: MIT Press.

Decety, J. & Wheatley, T. (2015, Eds.). *The moral brain: A multidisciplinary perspective.* Boston, MA: MIT Press.

den Houting, J. (2019). Neurodiversity: An insider's perspective. *Autism, 23*, 271–273.

Dozio, E., Feldman, M., Bizouerne, C., Drain, E., *et al.* (2020). The transgenerational transmission of trauma: The effects of maternal PTSD in mother-infant interactions. *Frontiers in Psychiatry, 11*, e480690.

Drack, M. (2015). Ludwig von Bertalanffy's organismic view on the theory of evolution. *Journal of Experimental Zoology. Part B, Molecular and Developmental Evolution, 324* (2), 77–90.

Elder, L.M., Dawson, G., Toth, K., Fein, D. & Munson, J. (2008). Head circumference as an early predictor of autism symptoms in younger siblings of children with autism spectrum disorder. *Journal of Autism and Developmental Disorders, 38* (6), 1104–1111.

Elwell, F. (2013). *Sociocultural systems: Principles of structure and change.* Edmonton, AB: AU Press.

Esbenson, A., Bishop, S., Mailick Seltzer, M., Greenberg, J.S. & Lounds Taylor, J. (2010). Comparisons between individuals with autism spectrum disorders and individuals with Down syndrome in adulthood. *American Journal of Intellectual Developmental Disabilities, 115* (4), 277–290.

Evans, C., Sanders, D. & Knight, R. (2014). 'LEGO Therapy' Club for children with high functioning autism and Asperger's syndrome. *Clinical Psychology Forum, 262*, 18–21.

Evans, V. & Bond, C. (2021). The implementation of LEGO®-Based Therapy in two English mainstream primary schools. *Journal of Research in Special Educational Needs, 21* (2), 111–119.

Farley, M., Cottle, J.K., Bilder, D., Viskochil, J., Coon, H. & McMahon, W. (2018). Mid-life social outcomes for a population-based sample of adults with ASD. *Autism Research, 11* (1), 142–152.

Farley, M., McMahon, W.M., Fombonne, E.W., Jenson, W.R., Miller, J., Gardner, M., Block, H., Pingree, C.B., Ritvo, R.A. & Coon, H. (2009). Twenty-year outcome for individuals with autism and average or near-average cognitive abilities. *Autism Research, 2* (2), 109–118.

Felin, T., Koslowski, S.W. & Chao, G.T. (2012). The dynamics of emergence: Cognition and cohesion in work teams. *Managerial and Decision Economics, 33*, 5–6.

Ferster, C.B. (1953). The use of the free operant in the analysis of behavior. *Psychological Bulletin, 50*, 263–274.

Ferster, C.B. (1961). Positive reinforcement and behavioral deficits of autistic children. *Child Development, 32*, 437–456.

Ferster, C.B. & DeMyer, M.K. (1961). The development of performances in autistic children in an automatically controlled environment. *Journal of Chronic Diseases, 13* (4), 312–345.

Fitch, W.T., Huber, L. & Bugnyar, T. (2010). Social cognition and the evolution of language: constructing cognitive phylogenies. *Neuron, 65* (6), 795–814.

Foley, R.A. & Lahr, M.M. (2011). The evolution of the diversity of cultures. *Philosophical Transactions of the Royal Society of London. Series B, Biological Sciences, 366* (1567), 1080–1089.

Frank, F., Jablotschkin, M., Arthen, T., Riedel, A., Fangmeier, T., Holzel, L.P. & van Elst, L.T. (2018). Education and employment status of adults with autism spectrum disorders in Germany—a cross-sectional survey. *BMC Psychiatry, 18* (75), 1–10.

Freud, S. (1938). *An outline of psychoanalysis.* London, UK: Hogarth.

Friston, K.J. (2010). The free-energy principle: A unified brain theory? *Nature Reviews Neuroscience, 11* (2), 127–138.

Friston, K.J., Lin, M., Frith, C.D., Pezzulo, G., Hobson, J.A. & Ondobaka, S. (2017). Active inference, curiosity, and insight. *Neural Computation, 29* (10), 2633–2683.

Friston, K.J. & Stephan, K. (2007). Free energy and the brain. *Synthese, 159* (3), 417–458.

Fuld, S. (2018). Autism Spectrum Disorder: The impact of stressful and traumatic life events and implications for clinical practice. *Clinical Social Work Journal, 46* (3), 210–219.

Gallo-Lopez & Rubin (Eds. 2011). (Eds.), *Play-Based Interventions for Children and Adolescents on the Autism Spectrum.* New York: Routledge Publishing.

Gaskins, S., Haight, W. & Lancy, D.F. (2006). The cultural construction of play. In, A. Göncü & S. Gaskins (Eds.). *Play and development: Evolutionary, sociocultural and functional perspectives*. Mahwah, NJ: Lawrence Erlbaum Associates, pp. 179–202.

Geary, D.C. (2005). *The origin of mind: Evolution of brain, cognition, and general intelligence*. Washington, DC: APA Press.

Georgiades, S., Szatmari, P., Zwaigenbaum, L., Bryson, S., Brian, J., Roberts, W., *et. al.* (2013). A prospective study of autistic-like traits in unaffected siblings of probands with autism spectrum disorder. *JAMA Psychiatry, 70* (1), 42–48.

Gibson, J.L., Pritchard, E. & de Lemos, C. (2021). Play-based interventions to support social and communication development in autistic children aged 2–8 years: A scoping review. *Autism & Developmental Language Impairments, 6*, 1–30.

Gilliam, J.E. (1995). *Gilliam autism rating scale (GARS)*. Austin, TX: Pro-Ed.

Ginsburg, K.R. and the Committee on Communications, and the Committee on Psychosocial Aspects of Child and Family Health (2007). The importance of play in promoting healthy child development and maintaining strong parent-child bonds. *Pediatrics, 119* (1), 181–191.

Göncü, A. (Ed). (1999). *Children's engagement in the world: Sociocultural perspectives*. New York, NY: Cambridge University Press.

Göncü, A. & Gaskins, S. (2006). *Play and development: Evolutionary, sociocultural and functional perspectives*. Mahwah, NJ: Lawrence Erlbaum Associates.

Göncü, A., Jain, J. & Teurmer, U. (2006). Children's play as cultural interpretation. In, A. Göncü & S. Gaskins (Eds.), *Play and development: Evolutionary, sociocultural and functional perspectives*. Mahwah, NJ: Lawrence Erlbaum Associates.

Goos, M., Galbraith, P. & Renshaw, P. (2002). Socially mediated metacognition: creating collaborative zones of proximal development in small group problem solving. *Educational Studies in Mathematics, 49*, 193–223.

Granqvist, P. (2021). Attachment, culture, and gene-culture co-evolution: expanding the evolutionary toolbox of attachment theory. *Attachment & Human Development, 23* (1), 90–113.

Green, J. (2020). Intervention during the prodromal stages of autism spectrum disorders. In, K. Chawarska, & F.R. Volkmar (Eds.), *Autism spectrum disorder in the first years of life: Research, assessment, and treatment*. Guilford Press, pp. 247–275.

Green, J., Aldred, C., Charman, T., Le Couteur, A., Emsley, R.A., Grahame, V., Howlin, P., Humphrey, N., Leadbitter, K., McConachie, H., Parr, J.R., Pickles, A., Slonims, V., Taylor, C. & PACT-G Group (2018). Paediatric Autism Communication Therapy-Generalised (PACT-G) against treatment as usual for reducing symptom severity in young children with autism spectrum disorder: Study protocol for a randomised controlled trial. *Trials, 19* (1), e514.

Green, J., Charman, T., McConachie, H., Aldred, C., Slonims, V., Howlin, P., Le Couteur, A., Leadbitter, K., Hudry, K., Byford, S., Barrett, B., Temple, K., Macdonald, W., Pickles, A. & PACT Consortium (2010). Parent-mediated communication-focused treatment in children with autism (PACT): A randomised controlled trial. *Lancet, 375* (9732), 2152–2160.

Green, J., Charman, T., Pickles, A., Wan, M.W., Elsabbagh, M., Slonims, V., *et al.* (2015). Parent-mediated intervention versus no intervention for infants at high risk of autism: A parallel, single-blind, randomised trial. *The Lancet Psychiatry, 2* (2), 133–140.

Green, J., Leadbitter, K., Ellis, C., Taylor, L., Moore, H.L., Carruthers, S., James, K., Taylor, C., *et al.* (2022). *An adapted social communication intervention at home and education to promote social communication changed in children with severe autism: The PACT-G RCT.* Southampton, UK: National Institute for Health Care Research.

Green, J., Pickles, A., Pasco, G., Bedford, R., Wan, M.W., Elsabbagh, M., *et al.* (2017). Randomised trial of a parent-mediated intervention for infants at high risk for autism: Longitudinal outcomes to age 3 years. *Journal of Child Psychology and Psychiatry, 58* (12), 1330–1340.

Green, J., Wan, M.W., Guiraud, J., Holsgrove, S., McNally, J., Slonims, V., *et al.* (2013). Intervention for infants at risk of developing autism: A case series. *Journal of Autism and Developmental Disorders, 43* (11), 2502–2514.

Griffiths, C. (2016). *LEGO therapy and social competence: An exploration of parental and teacher perceptions of LEGO-Based Therapy with pupils diagnosed with autism spectrum disorder (ASD).* Doctoral thesis in educational psychology, Cardiff University, Cardiff, Wales, UK.

Groh, A.M., Narayan, A.J., Bakermans-Kranenburg, M.J., Roisman, G.I., Vaughn, B.E., Pasco Fearon, R.M. & van Ijzendoorn, M.H. (2017). Attachment and temperament in the early life course: A meta-analytic review. *Child Development, 88* (3), 770–795.

Grzadzinski, R.L., Luyster, R., Spencer, A.G. & Lord, C. (2014). Attachment in young children with autism spectrum disorders: An examination of separation and reunion behaviors with both mothers and fathers. *Autism, 18* (2), 85–96.

Gunduz, N. & Hursen, C. (2015). Constructivism in teaching and learning; Content analysis evaluation. *Procedia: Social and Behavioral Sciences, 191*, 527–533.

Guo, Y., Garfin, D.R., Ly, A. & Goldberg, W.A. (2017). Emotion coregulation in mother-child dyads: A dynamic systems analysis of children with and without autism spectrum disorder. *Journal of Abnormal Child Psychology, 45* (7), 1369–1383.

Guralnick, M.J. (2019). *Effective early intervention: The developmental systems approach.* Baltimore, MD: Brookes Publishing.

Ha, T. (2022). Pretend play and early language development—relationships and impacts: A comprehensive literature review. *Journal of Education, 202* (1), 122–130.

Hamilton, W.D. (1964). The genetical evolution of social behavior, I & II. *Journal of Theoretical Biology, 7* (1), 1–52.

Harrison, P.L. & Oakland, T. (2015). *Adaptive Behavior Assessment System, Third Edition (ABAS-3).* Torrance, CA: Western Psychological Services.

Haxby, J.V., Hoffman, E.A. & Gobbini, M.I. (2002). Human neural systems for face recognition and social communication. *Biological Psychiatry, 51,* 59–67.

Hebb, D.O. (1949). *The organization of behavior: A neuropsychological theory.* New York, NY: Wiley & Sons.

Heninger, N.A. & Taylor, J.L. (2013). Outcome of adults with autism spectrum disorders: A historical perspective. *Autism, 17* (1), 103–116.

Herrington, J.D., Maddox, B.B., Kerns, C.M., Rump, K., *et al.* (2017). Amygdala volume differences in autism spectrum disorder are related to anxiety. *Journal of Autism and Developmental Disorders, 47* (12), 3682–3691.

Holtzstrom, J. & Anderson, H. (2021). Exploring and extending the synergy concept—A study of three acquisitions. *Journal of Business and Industrial Marketing, 36* (13), 28–41.

Howlin, P. & Moss, P. (2012). Adults with autism spectrum disorders. *The Canadian Journal of Psychiatry, 57* (5), 275–283.

Hu, X., Zheng, Q. & Lee, G.T. (2018). Using peer-mediated LEGO® Play intervention to improve social interactions for Chinese children with autism in an inclusive setting. *Journal of Autism and Developmental Disorders, 48* (7), 2444–2457.

Hughes, F.P. (2010). *Children, play and development.* Los Angeles, CA: Sage Publishing.

Hull, K.B. (2011). *Play therapy and Asperger's Syndrome: Helping children and adolescents grow, connect, and heal through the art of play.* Lanham, MD: Jason Aronson Publishing.

Hull, L., Levy, L., Lai, M.C., Petrides, K.V., Baron-Cohen, S., Allison, C., Smith, P. & Mandy, W. (2021). Is social camouflaging associated with anxiety and depression in autistic adults? *Molecular Autism, 12,* 13.

Huskens, B., Palmen, A., Van der Werff, M., Lourens, T. & Barakova, E. (2015). Improving collaborative play between children with autism spectrum disorders and their siblings: The effectiveness of a robot-mediated intervention based on LEGO® therapy. *Journal of Autism and Developmental Disorders, 45* (11), 3746–3755.

IDEA (2004). *Individuals with Disabilities Education Act*, 20 U.S.C. § 1400.

Johnson, S.C., Dweck, C.S., Chen, F.S., Ster, H.L., Ok, S.J. & Barth, M. (2010). At the intersection of social and cognitive development: Internal working models of attachment in infancy. *Cognitive Science, 34* (5) 807–825.

Jonsdottir, S.L., Brynjarsdottir, B., Saemundson, E. & Sigurdsson, J.F. (2018). Long-term outcome of children with autism who received different forms of early intervention during their preschool years: A pilot study of 15 young adults. *Scandinavian Journal of Child and Adolescent Psychiatry and Psychology, 6* (1), 28–39.

Kalso, E. (2011). The vicious circle in chronic pain management: Balancing efficacy and adverse effects. *Current Medical Research and Opinion, 27* (10), 2069–2071.

Kato, D., Hattori, K., Iwai, S. & Morita, M. (2012). Effects of collaborative expression using LEGO® blocks, on social skills and trust. *Social Behavior and Personality: An International Journal, 40* (7), 1195–1200.

Keenan, B.M., Newman, L.K., Gray, K.M. & Rinehart, N.J. (2016). Parents of children with ASD experience more psychological distress, parenting stress, and attachment-related anxiety. *Journal of Autism and Developmental Disorders, 46* (9), 2979–2991.

Keller, H. (2018). Universality claim of attachment theory: Children's socioemotional development across cultures. *Proceedings of the National Academy of Sciences of the United States of America, 115* (45), 11414–11419.

Keller, M.N. & Noone, R.J. (Eds., 2020). *Handbook of Bowen family systems theory and research methods: A systems model for family research.* New York, NY: Routledge Publishing.

Kellerman, A.M., Schwichtenberg, A.J., Tonnsen, B.L., Posada, G. & Lane, S.P. (2019). Dyadic interactions in children exhibiting the broader autism phenotype: Is the broader autism phenotype distinguishable from typical development? *Autism Research: Official Journal of the International Society for Autism Research, 12* (3), 469–481.

Kinkade, K. (1973). *A Walden Two experiment: The first five years of Twin Oaks Community.* New York, NY: William Morrow and Company.

Kirkham, J., Stewart, A., Kidd, E. (2013). Concurrent and longitudinal relationships between development in graphic, language and symbolic play domains from the fourth to the fifth year. *Infant and Child Development, 22* (3), 297–319.

Koeners, M.P. & Francis, J. (2020). The physiology of play: Potential relevance for higher education. *International Journal of Play, 9* (1), 143–159.

Kozlowski, S.W.J. & Chao, G.T. (2012). The dynamics of emergence: Cognition and cohesion in work teams. *Managerial & Decision Economics, 33*, 335–354.

Kozlowski, S.W., Chao, G.T., Grand, J.A., Braun, M.T. & Kuljanin, G. (2013). Advancing multilevel research design capturing the dynamics of emergence. *Organizational Research Methods, 16*, 581–615.

Kuhlmann, H. (2005). *Living Walden Two.* Chicago, IL: University of Illinois Press.

Kulju, L. & Mäki, E. (2017). *LEGO-Based Therapy supporting children's social participation in occupational therapy group: Occupational Therapist's handbook.* Oulu, Finland: Oulu University of Applied Sciences.

LaFreniere, P. (2011). Evolutionary functions of social play: Life histories, sex differences, and emotion regulation. *American Journal of Play, 3* (4), 464–488.

Laszlo, E. (1969). *System, structure, and experience: Toward a scientific theory of mind.* New York, NY: Gordon & Breach.

Laszlo, E. (1972a). *Introduction to systems philosophy: Toward a new paradigm of contemporary thought.* London, UK: Gordon & Breach Science.

Laszlo, E. (1972b). *The systems view of the world.* New York, NY: Braziller.

Latash, M. (2008). *Synergy.* New York, NY: Oxford University Press.

Latash, M. (2010). Motor synergies and the equilibrium-point hypothesis. *Motor Control, 14* (3), 294–322.

Latash, M. (2016). Towards physics of neural processes and behavior. *Neuroscience and Biobehavioral Reviews, 69*, 136–146.

Latash, M. (2021). Understanding and synergy: A single concept at different levels of analysis? *Frontiers in Systems Neuroscience, 15*, e735406.

Laughlin, P.R. & Barth, J.M. (1981). Group-to-individual and individual-to-group problem-solving transfer. *Journal of Personality and Social Psychology, 41* (6), 1087–1093.

Laughlin, P.R., Bonner, B.L. & Miner, A.G. (2002). Groups perform better than the best individuals on letters-to-numbers problems. *Organizational Behavior and Human Decision Processes, 88*, 605–620.

Laughlin, P.R., Carey, H.R. & Kerr, N.L. (2008). Group-to-Individual Problem-Solving Transfer. *Group Processes & Intergroup Relations, 11*(3), 319–330.

Laughlin, P.R., Hatch, E.C., Silver, J.S. & Boh, L. (2006). Groups perform better than the best individuals on letters-to-numbers problems: Effects of group size. *Journal of Personality and Social Psychology, 90*, 644–651.

Laughlin, P.R. & Sweeney, J.D. (1977). Individual-to-group and group-to-individual transfer in problem solving. *Journal of Experimental Psychology: Human Learning and Memory, 3* (2), 246–254.

Lawson, R.P., Mathys, C. & Rees, G. (2017). Adults with autism overestimate the volatility of the sensory environment. *Nature Neuroscience, 20* (9), 1293–1299.

Leadbitter, K., Buckle, K.L., Ellis, C. & Dekker, M. (2021). Autistic self-advocacy and the neurodiversity movement: Implications for autism early intervention research and practice. *Frontiers in Psychology, 10,* e3389.

LeGoff, D.B. (2004). Use of LEGO® as a therapeutic medium for improving social competence. *Journal of Autism and Developmental Disorders, 34* (5), 557–571.

LeGoff, D.B. (2017). *How LEGO®-based therapy works: Landing on my planet.* London, UK: Jessica Kingsley Publishers.

LeGoff, D.B. (2023). *Being autistic is not a behavior problem: A critique of applied behavior analysis the era of neurodiversity.* Universal Publishing: Boca Raton, FL.

LeGoff, D.B., Gomez de la Cuesta, G., Krauss, G.W. & Baron Cohen, S. (2014). *LEGO®-based therapy: How to build social competence through LEGO®-based clubs for children with autism and related conditions.* London, UK: Jessica Kingsley Publishers.

LeGoff, D.B., Krauss, G.W. & Allen, S. (2010). LEGO® play therapy for children with autistic disorders. In, A.A. Drewes & C.E. Schaefer (Eds), *School-Based Play Therapy, Second Edition.* Hoboken, NJ: John Wiley & Sons.

LeGoff, D.B., Krauss, G.W. & Allen, S.L. (2011). Innovative uses of LEGO® materials for improving social competence in children and adolescents. In, L. Gallo-Lopez, and L. Rubin, (Eds.), *Play-Based Interventions for Children and Adolescents on the Autism Spectrum.* New York: Routledge Publishing.

LeGoff, D.B. & Sherman, M. (2006). Long-term outcome of social skills intervention based on interactive LEGO® play. *Autism, 10* (4), 1–31.

Levy, J. & Dunsmuir, S. (2020). LEGO Therapy: Building social skills for adolescents with an autism spectrum disorder. *Educational & Child Psychology, 37* (1), 58–83.

Lewis, V., Boucher, J., Lupton, L., Watson, S. (2000). Relationships between symbolic play, functional play, verbal and non-verbal ability in young children. *International Journal of Language & Communication Disorders, 35,* 117–127.

Lindsay, S. (2017). Systematic review of factors affecting driving and motor vehicle transportation among people with autism spectrum disorder. *Disability Rehabilitation, 39* (9), 837–846.

Lindsay, S., Hounsell, K.G. & Cassiani, C. (2017). A scoping review of the role of LEGO® therapy for improving inclusion and social skills among children and youth with autism. *Disability and Health Journal, 10* (2), 173–182.

Liu, S., Solis, S., Jensen, H., Hopkins, E., Neale, D., Zosh, J. & Whitebread, D. (2017). *Neuroscience and learning through play: A review of the evidence* (research summary). Billund, DK: The LEGO Foundation.

Lorenz, E. (1963). Deterministic nonperiodic flow. *Journal of the Atmospheric Sciences, 2*0 (2), 130–141.

Lovaas, O.I. (1981). *Teaching developmentally disabled children: The ME book.* Baltimore, MD: University Park Press.

Lovaas, O.I. (1987). Behavioral treatment and normal educational and intellectual functioning in young autistic children. *Journal of Consulting and Clinical Psychology, 55*, 3–9.

Lovaas, O.I. (1993). The development of a treatment-research project for developmentally disabled and autistic children. *Journal of Applied Behavior Analysis, 26*, 617–630.

Lovaas, O.I., Koegel, R., Simmons, J. & Long, J. (1973). Some generalization and follow up measures on autistic children in behavior therapy. *Journal of Applied Behavior Analysis, 6*, 131–166.

Lovaas, O.I., Schreibman, L. & Koegel, R.L. (1974). A behavior modification approach to the treatment of autistic children. *Journal of Autism and Childhood Schizophrenia, 4*, 111–129.

Luria, A.R. (1973). *The working brain.* New York, NY: Basic Books.

Luria, A.R. (2002). L.S. Vygotsky and the problem of functional localization. *Journal of Russian and East European Psychology, 40*, 17–25.

MacCormack, J.W.H., Hutchinson, I.A. & Matheson, N.L. (2015). An exploration of a LEGO® based social skills program for youth with autism spectrum disorder. *Exceptionality Education International, 25*, 13–32.

Maitland, C.A., Rhodes, S., O'Hare, A. & Stewart, M.E. (2021). Social identities and mental well-being in autistic adults. *Autism: International Journal of Research and Practice, 25* (6), 1771–1783.

Martin, K.B., Haltigan, J.D., Ekas, N., Prince, E.B. & Messinger, D.S. (2020). Attachment security differs by later autism spectrum disorder: A prospective study. *Developmental Science, 27*, e12954.

MacDonald, H.Z., Beeghly, M., Grant-Knight, W., Augustyn, M., Woods, R.W., Cabral, H., Rose-Jacobs, R., Saxe, G.N. & Frank, D.A. (2008). Longitudinal association between infant disorganized attachment and childhood posttraumatic stress symptoms. *Development and Psychopathology, 20* (2), 493–508.

McEachin, J.J., Smith, T. & Lovaas, I.O. (1993). Long-term outcome for children with autism who received early intensive behavioral treatment. *American Journal on Mental Retardation, 97*, 359–372.

Meltzoff, A.N. (2002). Imitation as a mechanism of social cognition: Origins of empathy, theory of mind, and the representation of action. In, U. Goshwami (Ed.), *Blackwell handbook of childhood cognitive development.* London, UK: Blackwell Publishers.

Meltzoff, A.N. (2007). 'Like me,' a foundation for social cognition. *Developmental Science, 10*, 126–134.

Meltzoff, A.N. & Decety, J. (2003). What imitation tells us about social cognition: A rapprochement between developmental psychology and cognitive neuroscience. *Philosophical Transactions of the Royal Society of London, Biological Sciences, 358* (1431), 491–500.

Meltzoff, A.N., Kuhl, P.K., Movellan, J. & Sejnowski, T.J. (2009). Foundations for a new science of learning. *Science, 325*, 284–288.

Mesibov, G.B. (1992). Treatment issues with high-functioning adolescents and adults with autism. In, E. Schopler & G.B. Mesibov, Editors, *Social behavior in autism.* (pp. 265–230). New York, NY: Plenum Press.

Miron, A.M. & Brehm, J.W. (2006). Reactance theory—40 years later. *Zeitschrift fur Sozialpsychologie, 37* (1), 3–11.

Moll, H. & Tomasello, M. (2007). Cooperation and human cognition: The Vygotskian intelligence hypothesis. *Philosophical Transactions of the Royal Society of London: Biological Sciences, 362* (1480), 639–642.

Moody, C.T. & Laugeson, E.A. (2020). Social skills training in autism spectrum disorder across the lifespan. *Psychiatric Clinics of North America, 43* (4), 687–699.

Muentener, P., Herrig, E. & Schulz, L. (2018). The efficiency of infants' exploratory play is related to longer-term cognitive development. *Frontiers in Psychology, 9*, e635.

Muthukrishna, M. & Henrich, J. (2016). Innovation in the collective brain. *Philosophical Transactions of the Royal Society, Biological Sciences, 371*, 20150192.

Muthukrishna, M., Doebeli, M., Chudek, M. & Henrich, J. (2018). The Cultural Brain Hypothesis: How culture drives brain expansion, sociality, and life history. *PLoS Computational Biology 14*, (11), e1006504.

Myers, R.K., Bonsu, J.M., Carey, M.E., Yerys, B.E., Mollen, C.J. & Curry, A.E. (2019). Teaching autistic adolescents and young adults to drive: Perspectives of specialized driving instructors. *Autism in Adulthood: Challenges and Management, 1* (3), 202–209.

Narzisi, A., Sesso, G., Berloffa, S., Fontozzi, P., Muccio, R., Valente, E., Viglione, V., Villafranca, A., Milonee, A. & Masi, G. (2021). Could you give me the bluebrick? LEGO®-Based Therapy as a social development program for children with autism spectrum disorder: A systematic review. *Brain Sciences, 11*, 702.

Nguyen, C.T. (2016). *Sociality in autism: Building social bridges in autism spectrum conditions through LEGO®-based therapy.* Doctoral Thesis, University of Hertfordshire, Hatfield, UK.

Nijhof, S.L., Vinkers, C.H., van Geelan, S.M., Dujiff, S.N., Marijke Achterberg, E.J., *et al.* (2018). Healthy play, better coping: The importance of play for the development of children in health and disease. *Neuroscience & Biobehavioral Reviews, 95*, 421–429.

Ohl, A., Grice Sheff, M., Small, S., Nguyen, J., Paskor, K. & Zankirian, A. (2017). Predictors of employment status among adults with autism spectrum disorder. *Work, 56* (2), 345–355.

Owens, G., Granader, Y., Humphrey, A. & Baron Cohen, S. (2008). LEGO® therapy and the Social Use of Language Programme: An evaluation of two social skills interventions for children with high functioning autism and Asperger Syndrome. *Journal of Autism and Developmental Disorders, 38* (10), 1944–1957.

Ozonoff, S., Iosif, A., Baguio, F., Cook, I., Hill, M., Hutman, T., *et al.* (2010). A prospective study of the emergence of early behavioral signs of autism. *Journal of American Academy of Child Adolescent Psychiatry, 49* (3), 256–266.

Ozonoff, S., Young, G.S., Belding, A., Hill, M., Hill, A., Hutman, T., *et al.* (2014). The broader autism phenotype in infancy: When does it emerge? *Journal of the American Academy of Child & Adolescent Psychiatry, 53* (4), 398–407.

Pang, Y. (2010). LEGO games help young children with autism develop social skills. *International Journal of Education, 2* (2), E7.

Pavlov, I.P. (1927). *Conditioned reflexes: an investigation of the physiological activity of the cerebral cortex.* Oxford, UK: Oxford University Press.

Pavlov, I.P. (1941). *Conditioned reflexes and psychiatry.* London, UK: Lawrence & Wishart Press.

Peckett, H., MacCallum, F. & Knibbs, J. (2016). Maternal experience of LEGO-based therapy in families with children with autism spectrum conditions: What is the impact on family relationships? *Autism, 20*, 879–887.

Pellegrini, A.D. (2009). *The role of play in human development.* Oxford, UK: Oxford University Press.

Pellegrini, A.D. & Smith, P.K. (2008). The development of play during childhood: Forms and possible functions. *Child Psychology and Psychiatry Review, 3* (2), 51–57.

Pellegrini, A.D. & Smith, P.K. (1998). Physical activity play: The nature and function of a neglected aspect of play. *Child Development, 69* (3), 577–598.

Pellis, S. & Pellis, V. (2009). *The Playful Brain: Venturing to the Limits of Neuroscience.* Oneworld Publications: Oxford, UK.

Perone, S. & Simmering, V.R. (2017). Chapter Two—Applications of dynamic systems theory to cognition and development: New Frontiers. *Advances in Child Development and Behavior, 52*, 43–80.

Piaget, J. (1962a). *Comments on Vygotsky's critical remarks concerning "The Language and thought of the child," and "Judgment and reasoning in the child."* Cambridge, MA: The MIT Press.

Piaget, J. (1962b). *Play, dreams and imitation in childhood.* New York: Norton.

Piaget, J. & Inhelder, B. (1972). *The psychology of the child.* New York, NY: Basic Books.

Pinker, S. (2010). Colloquium paper: The cognitive niche: coevolution of intelligence, sociality, and language. *Proceedings of the National Academy of Sciences of the United States of America, 107* (2), 8993–8999.

Posar, A. & Visconti, P. (2019). Long-term outcome of autism spectrum disorder. *Turkish Archives of Pediatrics, 54* (4), 207–212.

Priest, J.B. (2021). *The science of family systems theory.* New York, NY: Routledge.

Ralph, D. & Rochester, J. (2016). *Building Language Using LEGO® Bricks: A Practical Guide.* London, UK: Jessica Kingsley Publishing.

Ramalho, N.C.P. & Sarmento, S.M.S. (2019). LEGO® Therapy as an intervention in autism spectrum disorders: An integrative literature review. *Revista CEFAC, 21* (2), 1–10.

Reichow, B. & Volkmar, F.R. (2010). Social skills interventions for individuals with autism: Evaluation for evidence-based practices within a best evidence synthesis framework. *Journal of Autism and Developmental Disorders, 40* (2), 149–166.

Reinhard, M.A., Dewald-Kaufmann, J., Wüstenberg, T., Musil, R., Barton, B.B., *et al.* (2020). The vicious circle of social exclusion and psychopathology: A systematic review of experimental ostracism research in psychiatric disorders. *European Archives of Psychiatry & Clinical Neuroscience, 270* (5), 521–532.

Robinson-Drummer, P.A., Opendak, M., Blomqvist, A., Chan, S., Tan, S., Delmer, C., *et al.* (2019). Infant trauma alters social buffering of threat learning: Emerging role of prefrontal cortex in preadolescence. *Frontiers in Behavioral Neuroscience, 13*, e00132.

Rutgers, A.H., Bakermans-Kranenburg, M.J., van Ijzendoorn, M.H. & van Berckelaer-Onnes, I.A. (2004). Autism and attachment: A meta-analytic review. *Journal of Child Psychology & Psychiatry, 45* (6), 1123–1134.

Rutter, M. (2000). Genetic studies of autism: From the 1970s into the millennium. *Journal of Abnormal Child Psychology, 28* (1), 3–14.

Salmons, J., Wilson, L. & Strang, K.D. (2009). Collaborative synergy and leadership in e-business. In, K.D. Strang (Ed.), *Handbook of research on electronic collaboration and organizational synergy*, Hershey, PA: Global, pp. 409–434.

Sander, D., Grafman, J. & Zalla, T. (2003). The human amygdala: An evolved system for relevance detection. *Reviews in Neuroscience, 14* (4), 303–316.

Sandoval-Norton, A.H. & Shkedy, G. (2019). How much compliance is too much compliance: Is long-term ABA therapy abuse? *Cogent Psychology, 6* (1), e1641258.

Sandoval-Norton, A.H., Shkedy, G. & Shkedy, D. (2021). Long-term ABA therapy is abusive: A response to Gorycki, Ruppel, and Zane. *Advances in Neurodevelopmental Disorders, 5*, 126–134.

Sapkota, T., Houkes, I. & Bosma, H. (2021). Vicious cycle of chronic disease and poverty: A qualitative study in present day Nepal. *International Health, 13* (1), 30–38.

Schreibman, L., Dawson, G., Stahmer, A.C., Landa, R., Rogers, S.J., McGee, G.G, Kasari, C., Ingersoll, B., Kaisser, A.P., Bruinsma, Y., McNerney, E., Wetherby, A. & Halladay, A. (2015). Naturalistic developmental behavioral interventions: Empirically validated treatments for autism spectrum disorder. *Journal of Autism and Developmental Disorders, 45*, 2411–2428.

Schumann, C.M., Barnes, C.C., Lord, C. & Courchesne, E. (2009). Amygdala enlargement in toddlers with autism related to severity of social and communication impairments. *Biological Psychiatry, 66* (10), 942–949.

Schumann, C.M., Bauman, M.D. & Amaral, D.G. (2011). Abnormal structure or function of the amygdala is a common component of neurodevelopmental disorders. *Neuropsychologia, 49* (4), 745–759.

Schumann, C.M., Hamstra, J., Goodlin-Jones, B.L., Lotspeich, L.J., Kwon, H., Buonocore, M.H., Lammers, C.R., Reiss, A.L. & Amaral, D.G. (2004). The amygdala is enlarged in children but not adolescents with autism: The hippocampus is enlarged at all ages. *The Journal of Neuroscience, 24* (28), 6392–6401.

Shvarts, A. & Bakker, A. (2019). The early history of the scaffolding metaphor: Bernstein, Luria, Vygotsky, and before. *Mind, Culture, & Activity, 26* (1), 4–23.

Silva, E.B., Filipini, R., Monteiro, C.B., Valenti, V.E., de Carvalho, S.M., Wajnsztejn, R., de Farias, M., Macedo, C.C. & de Abreu, L.C. (2013). The biopsychosocial processes in autism spectrum disorder. *International Archives of Medicine, 6* (1), e22.

Simic, G., Tkalcic, M., Vukic, V., Mulc, D., Spanic, E., Sagud, M., Olucha-Bordonau, F.E., Vuksic, M. & Hof, P.R. (2021). Understanding emotions: Origins and roles of the amygdala. *Biomolecules, 11*, 823.

Singha, S., Warr, M., Mishra, P. & Henriksen, D. (2020). Playing with creativity across the lifespan: A conversation with Dr. Sandra Russ. *Tech Trends, 27*, 1–5.

Siviy, S.M. (2016). A brain motivated to play: Insights into the neurobiology of playfulness. *Behaviour, 153* (6–7), 819–844.

Siviy, S.M. & Panskepp, J. (2011). In search of the neurobiological substrates for social playfulness in mammalian brains. *Neuroscience Biobehavioral Reviews, 35* (9), 1821–1830.

Skinner, B.F. (1938). *The behavior of organisms: An experimental analysis.* Cambridge, MA: B.F. Skinner Foundation Reprint Series.

Skinner, B.F. (1948). *Walden Two.* Chicago, IL: Macmillan Publishing.

Skinner, B.F. (1957). *Verbal behavior.* New York, NY: Appleton-Century-Crofts.

Skinner, B.F. (1966). *Contingencies of reinforcement.* New York, NY: Appleton-Century-Crofts.

Skinner, B.F. (1968). *The technology of teaching.* New York, NY: Appleton-Century-Crofts.

Skinner, B.F. (1978). *Reflections on behaviorism and society.* Englewood Cliffs, NJ: Prentice-Hall.

Skúladóttir, H., Gunnarsdóttir, T.J., Halldórsdóttir, S., Sveinsdóttir, H., Holden, J.E. & Björnsdóttir, A. (2020). Breaking the vicious circle: Experiences of people in chronic pain on the pain rehabilitation journey. *Nursing Open, 7* (5), 1412–1423.

Smallwood, J. (2013). Distinguishing *how* from *why* the mind wanders: A process-occurrence framework for self-generated mental activity. *Psychological Bulletin, 139* (3), 519–535.

Smallwood, J. & Schooler, J.W. (2006). The restless mind. *Psychological Bulletin, 132* (4), 946–958.

Smallwood, J. & Schooler, J.W. (2014). The science of mind wandering: Empirically navigating the stream of consciousness. *Annual Review of Psychology, 66* (1), 487–518.

Smith, K. & Kirby, S. (2008). Cultural evolution: Implications for understanding the human language faculty and its evolution. *Philosophical Transactions of the Royal Society of London. Series B, Biological Sciences, 363* (1509), 3591–3603.

Smith, P.K. (2006). Evolutionary foundations and functions of play: An overview. In, A. Göncü, & S. Gaskins (Eds.), *Play and development: Evolutionary, sociocultural and functional perspectives.* Mahwah, NJ: Lawrence Erlbaum Associates, pp. 21–50.

Solomon, C. (2020). Autism and employment: Implications for employers and adults with ASD. *Journal of Autism & Developmental Disorders, 50*, 209–217.

Someh, I., Shanks, G. & Davern, M. (2019). Reconceptualizing synergy to explain the value of business analytics systems. *Journal of Information Technology, 34* (4), 371–391.

Sosnowy, C., Silverman, C. & Shattuck, P. (2017). Parents' and young adults' perspectives on transition outcomes for young adults with autism. *Autism, 22*, 29–39.

Sparrow, S.S., Balla, D.A. & Cicchetti, D.V. (1984). *Vineland Adaptive Behavior Scales*, Circle Pines, MN: American Guidance Service.

Sparrow, S.S., Cicchetti, D.V. & Balla, D.A. (2005). *Vineland Adaptive Behavior Scales, Second Edition*. Circle Pines, MN: American Guidance Service.

Sparrow, S.S., Cicchetti, D.V. & Saulnier, C.A. (2016). *Vineland Adaptive Behavior Scales, Third Edition*. San Antonio, TX: Pearson.

Stagl, K.C., Burke, C.S., Salas, E. & Pierce, L. (2006). Team adaptation: Realizing team synergy. In C.S. Burke, L.G. Pierce, & E. Salas (Eds.), *Understanding adaptability: A prerequisite for effective performance within complex environments*. New York, NY: Elsevier, (pp. 117–141).

Strath, K. (2010). *Critical Review: Is LEGO therapy effective as a social skills intervention for children with autism spectrum disorder?* Master's Thesis in Communication Sciences, Speech-Language Pathology, School of Communication Sciences and Disorders, University of Western Ontario, London, Ontario, Canada.

Szatmari, P., Chawarska, K., Dawson, G., Georgiades, S., Landa, R., Lord, C., Messinger, D.S., Thurm, A. & Halladay, A. (2016). Prospective longitudinal studies of infant siblings of children with autism: Lessons learned and future directions. *Journal of the American Academy of Child and Adolescent Psychiatry, 55* (3), 179–187.

Thapar, A. & Rutter, M. (2021). Genetic advances in autism. *Journal of Autism and Developmental Disorders, 51* (12), 4321–4332.

Tomasello, M. (1996). Piagetian and Vygotskian approaches to language acquisition. *Human Development, 39*, 269–276.

Tomasello, M. (1999). *The cultural origins of human cognition*. Cambridge: MA: Harvard University Press.

Tomasello, M., Carpenter, M., Call, J., Behne, T. & Moll, H. (2005). Understanding and sharing intentions: The origins of cultural cognition. *Behavioral Brain Sciences, 28* (5), 675–691.

Toth, K., Munson, J., Meltzoff, A.N. & Dawson, G. (2006). Early predictors of communication development in young children with autism spectrum disorder:

Joint attention, imitation, and toy play. *Journal of Autism and Developmental Disorders, 36* (8), 993–1005.

Tsai, K.C. (2012). Play, imagination, and creativity: A brief literature review. *Journal of Education and Learning, 1* (2), 15.

Tsai, H.W.J., Cebula, K. & Fletcher-Watson, S. (2017). The role of the broader autism phenotype and environmental stressors in the adjustment of siblings of children with autism spectrum disorders in Taiwan and the United Kingdom. *Journal of Autism and Developmental Disorders, 47* (8), e2363.

Turati, C., Natale, E. Bolognini, N., Senna, I., Picozzi, M., Longhi, E. & Macchi Cassia, V. (2013). The early development of human mirror mechanisms: Evidence from electromyographic recordings at 3 and 6 months. *Developmental Science, 12066.*

Vanderschuren, L.J., Achterberg, E.J. & Trezza, V. (2016). The neurobiology of social play and its rewarding value in rats. *Neuroscience and Biobehavioral Reviews, 70,* 86–105.

van IJzendoorn, M.H., Rutgers, A.H., Bakermans-Kranenburg, M.J., Swinkels, S.H.N., van Daalen, E., Dietz, C., Naber, F.B.A., Buitelaar, J.K. & van Engeland, H. (2007). Parental sensitivity and attachment in children with autism spectrum disorder: Comparison with children with mental retardation, with language delays, and with typical development. *Child Development, 78* (2), 597–608.

van Schaik, C.P. & Burkhart, J.M. (2011). Social learning and evolution: The cultural intelligence hypothesis. *Philosophical Transactions of the Royal Society of London: Biological Sciences, 366* (1567), 1008–1016.

van Schaik, C.P., Deaner, R.O. & Merrill, M.Y. (1999). The conditions for tool use in primates: Implications for the evolution of material culture. *Journal of Human Evolution, 36* (6), 719–741.

Verkuyten, M. & Killen, M. (2021). Tolerance, dissenting beliefs, and cultural diversity. *Child Development Perspectives, 15* (1), 51–56.

von Bertalanffy, K.L. (1934). Theoretische biologie [Theoretical biology]. *Philosophical Review, 43* (4), 417–420.

von Bertalanffy, K.L. (1950). An outline for General Systems Theory. *British Journal for the Philosophy of Science, 1* (2).

von Bertalanffy, K.L. (1968a). *General System Theory: Foundations, development, applications.* New York: George Brazillier.

von Bertalanffy, K.L. (1968b). *Organismic psychology theory.* Barre, MA: Clark University Barre Publishers.

Vygotsky, L.S. (1967). Play and its role in the mental development of the child. *Soviet Psychology, 5,* 6–18.

Vygotsky, L.S. (1934/1986). *Thought and Language.* Cambridge, MA: The MIT Press.

Vygotsky, L.S. (1933/1978). *Mind in society: The development of higher psychological processes.* Cambridge, MA: Harvard University Press.

Wadsworth, B.J. (2004). *Piaget's theory of cognitive and affective development: Foundations of constructivism (5th Edition).* Boston, MA: Allyn & Bacon Classics.

Wah, A. (2020). Cognitive processes underlying play and pretend play: A comparative cross-species study on degrees of memory, perception, imagination, and consciousness. *American Journal of Play, 12* (2), 156–177.

Wainryb, C., Shaw, L.A., Langley, M. & Cottam, K. (2004). Children's thinking about diversity of belief in the early school years: Judgments and relativism, tolerance, and disagreeing persons. *Child Development, 75* (3), 687–703.

Wainryb, C., Shaw, L.A. & Maianu, C. (1998). Tolerance and intolerance: Children's and adolescents' judgments of dissenting beliefs, speech, persons, and conduct. *Child Development, 69* (6), 1541–55.

Wang, S. & Aamodt, S. (2012). Play, stress, and the learning brain. *Cerebrum: The Dana Forum on Brain Science, 12.*

Wartini-Twardowska, J. & Twardowski, Z. (2019). Searching for synergy from a combination of heterogeneous business models: Measurement and assessment from the polish software industry. *Heliyon, 5* (7), e01970.

Webb, S.J. & Jones, E.J. (2009). Early identification of autism: Early characteristics, onset of symptoms, and diagnostic stability. *Infants and Young Children, 22* (2), 100–118.

Weir, E., Allison, C., Warrier, V. & Baron Cohen, S. (2021a). Increased prevalence of non-communicable physical health conditions among autistic adults. *Autism: The International Journal of Research and Practice, 25* (3), 681–694.

Weir, E., Allison, C., Ong, K. K. & Baron-Cohen, S. (2021b). An investigation of the diet, exercise, sleep, BMI, and health outcomes of autistic adults. *Molecular Autism, 12* (1), e31.

Whitebread, D., Neale, D., Jensen, H., Liu, C., Solis, S.L., Hopkins, E., Hirsh-Pasek, K. & Zosh, J. (2017). *The role of play in children's development: A review of the evidence.* Billund, DK: LEGO Foundation.

Whitehouse, A.J.O. (2017). Elizabeth Usher Memorial Lecture: Rethinking the clinical pathway for autism spectrum disorder and challenging the status quo. *International Journal of Speech-Language Pathology, 19* (3), 208–217.

Whitehouse, A.J.O., Varcin, K.J., Alvares, G.A., Barbaro, J., Bent, C., Boutrus, M., *et al.* (2019). Pre-emptive intervention versus treatment as usual for infants showing early behavioural risk signs of autism spectrum disorder: A single-blind, randomised controlled trial. *The Lancet: Child & Adolescent Health, 3* (9), 605–615.

Whitehouse, A.J.O., Varcin, K.J. & Pillar, S. (2021). Effect of preemptive intervention on developmental outcomes among infants showing early signs of autism: A randomized clinical trial of outcomes to diagnosis. *JAMA Pediatrics, 175* (11), e213298.

Whiten, A. & van Schaik, C.P. (2007). The evolution of animal 'cultures,' and social intelligence. *Philosophical Transactions of the Royal Society of London: Biological Sciences, 362* (1480), 603–620.

Wilson, N. J., Lee, H. C., Vaz, S., Vindin, P. & Cordier, R. (2018). Scoping review of the driving behaviour of and driver training programs for people on the autism spectrum. *Behavioural Neurology,* e6842306.

Winnicott, D.W. (1965). *Maturational processes and the facilitating environment: Studies in the theory of emotional development.* Madison, CT: International Universities Press.

Winston, R. & Chicot, R. (2016). The importance of early bonding on the long-term mental health and resilience of children. *London Journal of Primary Care, 8* (1), 12–14.

Wood, D.J., Bruner, J.S. & Ross, G. (1976). The role of tutoring in problem solving. *Journal of Child Psychiatry and Psychology, 17* (2), 89–100.

Wood, J.J., Drahota, A., Sze, K., Har, K., Chiu, A. & Langer, D.A. (2009). Cognitive behavioral therapy for anxiety in children with autism spectrum disorders: A randomized, controlled trial. *Journal of Child Psychology and Psychiatry, and Allied Disciplines, 50* (3), 224–234.

World Health Organization (2019). *International statistical classification of diseases and related health problems (10th Ed).* Geneva, Switzerland: WHO Press.

Wright, B., Gomez de la Cuesta, G., Varley, D. & LeGoff, D.B. (2017). *Manual for delivery of LEGO-based therapy for the I-SOCIALISE Randomized Controlled Trial (RCT), Version 1.0.* York, UK: York University.

Yalamanchili, M. (2015). *Effects of a LEGO® Intervention on Social Skills in Kindergarten Children with Autism Spectrum Disorders.* Ph.D. Thesis, Philadelphia College of Osteopathic Medicine, Philadelphia, PA, USA.

Zalla, T. & Sperduti, M. (2013). The amygdala and the relevance detection theory of autism: An evolutionary perspective. *Frontiers in Human Neuroscience, 7,* 894.

Zwaigenbaum, L., Bauman, M., Stone, W. L., Yirmiya, N., Estes, A., Hansen, R., *et al.* (2015). Early identification of Autism Spectrum Disorder: Recommendations for practice and research. *Pediatrics, 1* (36), 10–40.

www.ingramcontent.com/pod-product-compliance
Lightning Source LLC
Chambersburg PA
CBHW071714170526
45165CB00005B/2014